2nd edition
High-Yield Embryology

2nd edition
High-Yield Embryology

Ronald W. Dudek, Ph.D.

Full Professor

Department of Anatomy and Cell Biology

East Carolina University

Brody School of Medicine

Greenville, North Carolina

LIPPINCOTT WILLIAMS & WILKINS

A **Wolters Kluwer** Company

Philadelphia · Baltimore · New York · London
Buenos Aires · Hong Kong · Sydney · Tokyo

Editor: Elizabeth Nieginski
Editorial Director of Development: Julie P. Scardiglia
Development Editors: Marjory I. Fraser and Rosanne Hallowell
Managing Editor: Marette Magargle-Smith
Illustrator: Precision Graphics
Marketing Manager: Kelly Ray

351 West Camden Street
Baltimore, Maryland 21201-2436 USA

530 Walnut Street
Philadelphia, Pennsylvania 19106 USA

The publisher is not responsible (as a matter of product liability, negligence, or otherwise) for any injury resulting from any material contained herein. This publication contains information relating to general principles of medical care which should not be construed as specific instructions for individual patients. Manufacturers' product information and package inserts should be reviewed for current information, including contraindications, dosages, and precautions.

Printed in the United States of America

Library of Congress Cataloging-in-Publication Data

Dudek, Ronald W., 1950–.
  High-yield embryology / Ronald W. Dudek.—2nd ed.
    p. ; cm.
  Includes index.
  ISBN 0-7817-2132-6
  1. Embryology, Human—Outlines, syllabi, etc.   I. Title.
  [DNLM: 1. Embryology—Examination Questions.   2. Embryology—Outlines.   3. Fetal Development—
Examination Questions.   4. Fetal Development—Outlines.   QS 618.2 D845h 2000]
  QM601 .D83 2000
  612.6′4′0076—dc21   00-059359

The publishers have made every effort to trace the copyright holders for borrowed material. If they have inadvertently overlooked any, they will be pleased to make the necessary arrangements at the first opportunity.

We'd like to hear from you! If you have comments or suggestions regarding this Lippincott Williams & Wilkins title, please contact us at the appropriate customer service number listed below, or send correspondence to **book_comments@lww.com.** If possible, please remember to include your mailing address, phone number, and a reference to the book title and author in your message. To purchase additional copies of this book call our customer service department at **(800) 638-3030** or fax orders to **(301) 824-7390.** International customers should call **(301) 714-2324.**

00 01 02

1 2 3 4 5 6 7 8 9 10

Dedication

I would like to dedicate this book to my father, Stanley J. Dudek, who died Sunday, March 20, 1988, at 11 A.M. It was his hard work and sacrifice that allowed me access to the finest educational institutions in the country. It was by hard work and sacrifice that he showed his love for his wife, Lottie; daughter, Christine; and grandchildren, Karolyn, Jeannie, and Katie. I remember my father as a good man who did the best he could. He is missed and remembered.

Contents

Preface

The topic of embryology is increasingly represented on the USMLE Step 1 examination not only in the form of "pure" embryology questions, but also as part and parcel of clinical vignette questions related to the other basic sciences. Clinical vignette questions often blend embryology with pathology, genetics, clinical medicine, and, to a lesser extent, molecular biology. Because of this changing approach in the USMLE, and also in response to students' comments about the first edition of *High-Yield*™ Embryology, I have added a significant amount of new material to the second edition, as follows:

- Radiographs, magnetic resonance images, and photos of many congenital malformations have been added, along with their pathology as it relates to embryological development and clinical findings.
- There are new chapters on genetic diseases (Chapters 22–Numerical Chromosomal Abnormalities; Chapter 23–Structural Chromosomal Abnormalities; and Chapter 24–Single Gene Inherited Diseases). These chapters address all of the genetic diseases frequently included on the USMLE, including Down syndrome, Prader-Willi syndrome, Angelman syndrome, and Huntington disease.
- A chapter on pregnancy (Chapter 21) addresses the clinical features of the pregnant woman vis-à-vis embryological development, including prenatal diagnostic procedures.
- A chapter on teratology (Chapter 26) addresses various infectious agents and categories of drugs that are contraindicated during pregnancy, along with their sequelae.
- Genes and protein factors that are commonly known to play a major role in embryological development of various systems have been included where appropriate.

I think you will be pleasantly surprised to find that *High-Yield*™ Embryology, 2nd edition, covers all of the topics that are highly likely to appear on the USMLE Step 1, and presents these topics in a format conducive to answering the integrated and blended questions on the exam. After taking the USMLE Step 1, you are welcome to e-mail me at *dudekr@mail.ecu.edu* to convey any comments or suggestions, or to indicate any area that was particularly represented on the exam.

Ronald W. Dudek, Ph.D.

1

Prefertilization Events

I. GAMETES (oocytes and spermatozoa), descendants of **primordial germ cells,** are produced in the adult by either **oogenesis** or **spermatogenesis,** processes that involve **meiosis.** Primordial germ cells originate in the **wall of the yolk sac** of the embryo and migrate into the gonad region.

II. MEIOSIS (Figure 1-1), which occurs **only during the production of gametes,** consists of two cell divisions **(meiosis I and meiosis II)** and results in the formation of four gametes containing 23 chromosomes and 1N amount of DNA **(23,1N).** Meiosis:

    A. Reduces the number of chromosomes within the gametes to ensure that the human species number of chromosomes (46) can be maintained from one generation to another

    B. Redistributes maternal and paternal chromosomes to ensure genetic variability

    C. Promotes the exchange of small amounts of maternal and paternal DNA via **crossover** during meiosis I

III. FEMALE GAMETOGENESIS (OOGENESIS; Table 1-1)

    A. Primordial germ cells (46,2N) arrive in the ovary at week 4 of embryonic development and differentiate into **oogonia (46,2N).**

    B. Oogonia enter **meiosis I** and undergo DNA replication to form **primary oocytes (46,4N).** All primary oocytes are formed by the **fifth month of fetal life** and remain dormant in **prophase (diplotene) of meiosis I until puberty.**

    C. During a woman's ovarian cycle, a primary oocyte completes meiosis I to form a **secondary oocyte (23,2N)** and a **first polar body,** which probably degenerates.

    D. The secondary oocyte enters **meiosis II,** and ovulation occurs when the chromosomes align at metaphase. The secondary oocyte remains **arrested in metaphase of meiosis II** until fertilization occurs.

    E. At fertilization, the secondary oocyte completes meiosis II to form a **mature oocyte (23,1N)** and a **second polar body.**

IV. HORMONAL CONTROL OF THE FEMALE REPRODUCTIVE CYCLE (Figure 1-2)

    A. The hypothalamus secretes **gonadotropin releasing hormone (GNRH).**

    B. In response to GNRH, the adenohypophysis secretes the gonadotropins **follicle-stimulating hormone (FSH)** and **luteinizing hormone (LH).**

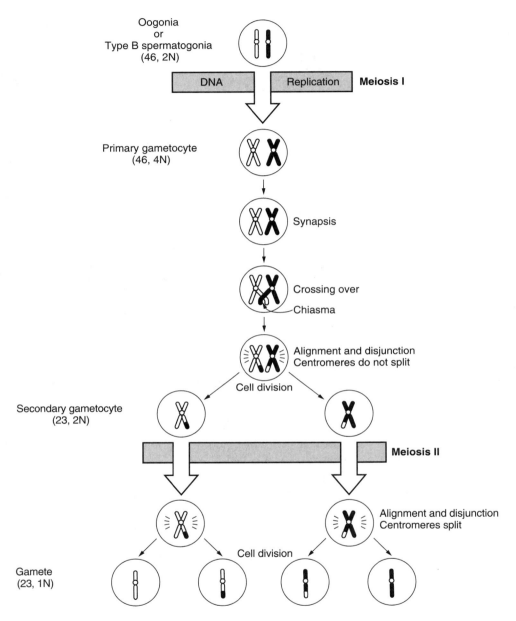

Figure 1-1. Schematic representation of meiosis I and meiosis II, emphasizing the chromosomal changes and amount of DNA that occur during either oogenesis or spermatogenesis. Note that only one pair of homologous chromosomes is shown (*white* = maternal origin; *black* = paternal origin). **Synapsis** is the process of pairing of homologous chromosomes. The point at which the DNA molecule crosses over is called the **chiasma,** which is where the exchange of small amounts of maternal and paternal DNA occur. Note that synapsis and crossing over occur only during meiosis I. (Adapted from Dudek RW, Fix JD: *BRS Embryology,* 2nd ed. Baltimore, Williams & Wilkins, 1998, p 4.)

Table 1-1
Number of Chromosomes and Amount of DNA Contained in Cells
During the Stage of Gametogenesis

Cell Type	No. of Chromosomes, Amount of DNA
Primordial germ cell, oogonia, spermatogonia (type A and B), zygote, blastomeres, all normal somatic cells	46, 2N
Primary oocyte, primary spermatocyte	46, 4N
Secondary oocyte, secondary spermatocyte	23, 2N
Oocyte (ovum), spermatid, sperm	23, 1N

    C. FSH stimulates the development of a secondary follicle to a graafian follicle within the ovary.

    D. Granulosa cells of the secondary and graafian follicle secrete **estrogen.**

    E. Estrogen stimulates the endometrium of the uterus to enter the **proliferative phase.**

    F. LH stimulates **ovulation.**

    G. Following ovulation, granulosa lutein cells of the corpus luteum secrete **progesterone.**

    H. Progesterone stimulates the endometrium of the uterus to enter the **secretory phase.**

V. MALE GAMETOGENESIS (SPERMATOGENESIS; see Table 1-1) is classically divided into three phases: spermatocytogenesis, meiosis, and spermiogenesis.

    A. Spermatocytogenesis

        1. **Primordial germ cells (46,2N)** arrive in the testes at week 4 of embryonic development and remain dormant until puberty. At puberty, primordial germ cells differentiate into **type A spermatogonia (46,2N).**

        2. Type A spermatogonia undergo **mitosis** to provide a continuous supply of stem cells throughout the reproductive life of the male (called **spermatocytogenesis**). Some type A spermatogonia differentiate into **type B spermatogonia (46,2N).**

    B. Meiosis

        1. Type B spermatogonia enter meiosis I and undergo DNA replication to form **primary spermatocytes (46,4N).**

        2. Primary spermatocytes complete meiosis I to form two **secondary spermatocytes (23,2N).**

        3. Secondary spermatocytes complete meiosis II to form four **spermatids (23,1N).**

    C. Spermiogenesis

        1. Spermatids undergo a **postmeiotic series of morphologic changes** (called spermiogenesis) to form **sperm (23,1N).** These changes include formation of the acrosome; condensation of the nucleus; and formation of the head, neck, and tail. The total time for sperm formation is approximately 64 days.

        2. Newly ejaculated sperm are incapable of fertilization until they undergo **capacitation,** which occurs in the female reproductive tract and involves the unmasking of sperm glycosyltransferases and removal of proteins that coat the surface of the sperm.

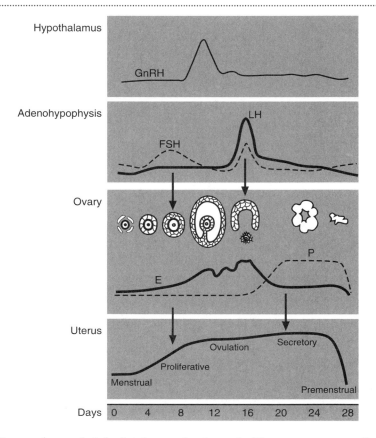

Figure 1-2. **Hormonal control of the female reproductive cycle.** The various patterns of hormone secretion from the hypothalamus, adenohypophysis, and ovary are shown. These hormones prepare the endometrium of the uterus for implantation of a conceptus. The menstrual cycle of the uterus consists of five phases. (1) The **menstrual phase** (days 1–4) is characterized by the **necrosis and shedding** of the functional layer of the endometrium. (2) The **proliferative phase** (days 4–15) is characterized by the **regeneration** of the functional layer of the endometrium and a **low basal body temperature** (97.5°F). (3) The **ovulatory phase** (days 14–16) is characterized by **ovulation** of a secondary oocyte and coincides with the surge in luteinizing hormone. (4) The **secretory phase** (days 15–25) is characterized by **secretory activity** of the endometrial glands and an **elevated basal body temperature** (over 98°F); implantation of a conceptus occurs in this phase. (5) The **premenstrual phase** (days 25–28) is characterized by **ischemia** due to reduced blood flow to the endometrium. E = estrogen; FSH = follicle-stimulating hormone; LH = luteinizing hormone; $GNRH$ = gonadotropin releasing hormone; P = progesterone. (From Dudek RW: *High-Yield Histology*, 2nd ed. Philadelphia, Lippincott Williams & Wilkins, 2000, p 170.)

VI. CLINICAL CORRELATIONS

A. Offspring of older women

1. **Prolonged dormancy of primary oocytes** may be the reason for the **high incidence of chromosomal abnormalities** in the offspring of older women. All primary oocytes are formed by the fifth month of fetal life; thus, a female infant is born with her entire supply of gametes. Primary oocytes remain dormant until ovulation. Oocytes that ovulated late in the woman's reproductive life may have been dormant for as long as 40 years.

2. The **incidence of trisomy 21 (Down syndrome) increases** with the advanced age of the mother.

B. **Offspring of older men.** An increased incidence of **achondroplasia** (a congenital skeletal anomaly characterized by retarded bone growth) is associated with advanced paternal age.

C. **Male fertility** depends on **the number and motility of sperm.** Fertile males produce from 20 to more than 100 million sperm/ml of semen. Sterile males produce less than 10 million sperm/ml of semen. Normally up to 10% of sperm in an ejaculate may be grossly deformed (two heads or two tails), but these sperm probably do not fertilize an oocyte owing to their lack of motility.

D. **Hormonal contraception**

    1. **Oral contraceptives**

        a. **Combination pills** contain a combination of **estrogen and progesterone.**

            (1) They are taken for 21 days and then discontinued for 7 days.

            (2) The primary mechanism of action is the inhibition of GNRH, FSH, and LH secretion, which prevents ovulation.

        b. **Progesterone-only pills** contain only progesterone.

            (1) They are taken continuously.

            (2) The primary mechanism of action is not known; however, progesterone-only pills cause thickening of cervical mucus, which makes is hostile to sperm migration, and thinning of the endometrium, which causes it to be unprepared for conceptus implantation.

    2. **Medroxyprogesterone acetate (Depo-Provera)** is a **progesterone-only** product that offers a **long-acting** alternative to oral contraceptives. It can be injected **intramuscularly** and will prevent ovulation for **2–3 months.**

    3. **Levonorgestrel (Norplant)** is a progesterone-only product that offers an even longer-acting alternative to oral contraceptives. The capsules containing levonorgestrel can be **implanted subdermally** and will prevent ovulation for **1–5 years.**

    4. **Luteinizing hormone releasing hormone (LHRH) analogues.** Chronic treatment with an LHRH analogue (e.g., **buserelin**) results paradoxically in a downregulation of FSH and LH secretion, thereby preventing ovulation.

    5. **Postcoital contraception ("morning-after pill")** can be used after unprotected intercourse.

        a. **Dosage.** Diethylstilbestrol (DES; 25 mg) is taken twice a day for 5 days; or, two combination pills are taken up to 72 hours after intercourse followed by two pills 12 hours later

        b. **Mechanism of action.** The high doses of steroids disrupt the endometrium so that implantation may not occur.

        c. **Precaution.** Because of the **potential teratogenic effects** of steroids, a therapeutic abortion is recommended if postcoital contraception fails and pregnancy occurs.

E. **Anovulation** is the absence of ovulation in some women owing to inadequate secretion of FSH and LH. This condition is often treated with **clomiphene citrate.** By competing with estrogen for binding sites in the adenohypophysis, clomiphene citrate suppresses the normal negative feedback loop of estrogen on the adenohypophysis. This in turn stimulates FSH and LH secretion and induces ovulation.

2
Week 1 (Days 1–7)*

I. OVERVIEW. Figure 2-1 summarizes the events that occur during week 1, following fertilization.

II. FERTILIZATION occurs in the **ampulla of the uterine tube.**

   A. The sperm binds to the zona pellucida of the secondary oocyte and triggers the **acrosome reaction,** causing the release of acrosomal enzymes (e.g., **acrosin**).

   B. Aided by the acrosomal enzymes, the sperm penetrates the zona pellucida. Penetration of the zona pellucida elicits the **cortical reaction,** rendering the secondary oocyte **impermeable to other sperm.**

   C. The sperm and secondary oocyte cell membranes fuse, and the contents of the sperm enter the cytoplasm of the oocyte.

   1. The male genetic material forms the **male pronucleus.**

   2. The tail and mitochondria of the sperm degenerate. Therefore, all mitochondria within the zygote are of maternal origin (i.e., **all mitochondrial DNA is of maternal origin**).

   D. The secondary oocyte completes meiosis II, thus forming a mature **ovum.** The nucleus of the ovum is the **female pronucleus.**

   E. The male and female pronuclei fuse to form a **zygote.**

III. CLEAVAGE is a series of **mitotic** divisions of the zygote.

   A. The zygote cytoplasm is successively cleaved to form a **blastula,** which consists of increasingly smaller **blastomeres** (e.g., the first blastomere stage consists of two cells; the next, four cells; the next, eight cells).

   B. At the 32-cell stage, the blastomeres form a **morula,** which consists of an **inner cell mass** and **outer cell mass.**

   C. Blastomeres are considered **totipotent** up to the eight-cell stage (i.e., each blastomere can form a complete embryo by itself, which is important when considering monozygotic twinning).

---

*The age of the developing conceptus can measured either from the estimated day of fertilization (**fertilization age**) or from the day of the **last normal menstrual period** (**LNMP**). In this book, ages are presented as fertilization age.

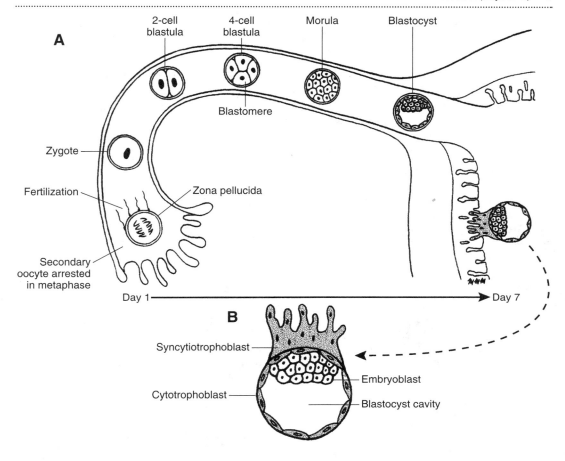

Figure 2-1.   (A) The stages of human development during week 1. (B) A blastocyst on day 7.

IV. **BLASTOCYST FORMATION** occurs when fluid secreted within the morula forms the
    blastocyst cavity.

   A. The inner cell mass, which becomes the **embryo,** is now called the **embryoblast.**

   B. The outer cell mass, which becomes part of the **placenta,** is now called the **trophoblast.**

V. **IMPLANTATION**

   A. The **zona pellucida must degenerate** for implantation to occur.

   B. The blastocyst implants within the **posterior superior wall** of the uterus. During the
   secretory phase of the menstrual cycle, the blastocyst implants within the **functional
   layer of the endometrium**

   C. The trophoblast differentiates into the **cytotrophoblast** and **syncytiotrophoblast.**

VI. **CLINICAL CORRELATIONS**

   A. Ectopic tubal pregnancy

1. This type of pregnancy occurs when the blastocyst implants within the uterine tube owing to **delayed transport.**

2. The **ampulla of uterine tube** is the **most common site** of an ectopic pregnancy. The **rectouterine pouch (pouch of Douglas)** is a common site for an ectopic abdominal pregnancy.

3. Ectopic pregnancy is most commonly seen in women with **endometriosis** or **pelvic inflammatory disease.**

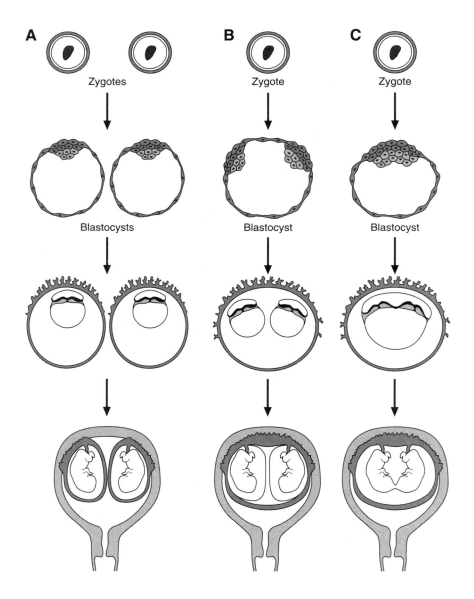

Figure 2-2. Diagram of twinning. (A) Dizygotic twins. (B) Monozygotic twins. (C) Conjoined twins.

4. **Uterine tube rupture and hemorrhage** may occur if surgical intervention (i.e., salpingectomy) is not performed.

5. An ectopic tubal pregnancy **presents with abnormal uterine bleeding and unilateral pelvic pain,** which must be differentially diagnosed from appendicitis, an aborting intrauterine pregnancy, or a bleeding corpus luteum of a normal intrauterine pregnancy.

B. Twinning (**Figure 2-2**)

1. **Dizygotic (fraternal) twins** result from the fertilization of two different secondary oocytes by two different sperm. The resultant two zygotes form two blastocysts, each of which implants separately into the endometrium of the uterus. Thus, these twins are no more genetically alike than are siblings born at different times.

2. **Monozygotic (identical)** result from the fertilization of one secondary oocyte by one sperm. The resultant zygote forms a blastocyst in which the inner cell mass (embryoblast) splits into two. Therefore, the twins are genetically identical.

3. **Conjoined (Siamese) twins.** In these monozygotic twins, the inner cell mass (embryoblast) does not completely split. The two embryos are joined by a tissue bridge (e.g., at the head, thorax, or pelvis).

C. **In vitro fertilization (Figure 2-3)** requires the sequential application of several of the following techniques.

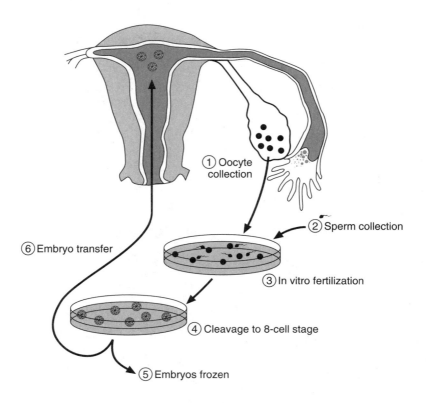

Figure 2-3.　Diagram of various steps involved with in vitro fertilization.

1. Clomiphene citrate is administered to stimulate multiple ovulation.

2. Oocytes are collected by needle aspiration from the ovary with the assistance of ultrasound visualization.

3. Sperm are collected via masturbation; the sperm are separated from seminal fluid and undergo capacitation by exposure to ionic solutions. In cases of oligospermia (infertility due to a low number of sperm), multiple samples may be obtained over an extended period of time.

4. Sperm and oocytes are cultured together. The success of in vitro fertilization is judged by the presence of two pronuclei with the oocyte.

5. Cleavage is allowed to proceed in vitro to the eight cell stage embryo.

6. Typically, at least three embryos are transferred to the uterus, because there is a low success rate of implantation.

7. The remaining embryos are frozen for future use in case the first embryo transfer does not result in a pregnancy.

3
Week 2 (Days 8–14)

I. EMBRYOBLAST (Figure 3-1). The embryoblast differentiates into two distinct cell layers, the **epiblast** and **hypoblast,** forming a **bilaminar embryonic disk.**

   A. Epiblast. Clefts develop within the epiblast to form the **amniotic cavity.**

   B. Hypoblast cells migrate along the cytotrophoblast, forming the **yolk sac.**

   C. The **prochordal plate,** formed by the fusion of epiblast and hypoblast cells, marks the future site of the **mouth.**

II. TROPHOBLAST

   A. The syncytiotrophoblast continues its growth into the endometrium to make contact with endometrial blood vessels and glands.

   1. The syncytiotrophoblast **does not divide mitotically.**

   2. The syncytiotrophoblast produces **human chorionic gonadotropin (HCG).**

   B. The cytotrophoblast does divide mitotically, adding to the growth of the syncytiotrophoblast. **Primary chorionic villi** protrude into the syncytiotrophoblast.

III. EXTRAEMBRYONIC MESODERM is a new layer of cells derived from the epiblast.

   A. Extraembryonic somatic mesoderm (somatopleuric mesoderm) lines the cytotrophoblast, forms the **connecting stalk,** and covers the amnion (see Figure 3-1).

   1. The conceptus is suspended by the connecting stalk within the **chorionic cavity.**

   2. The wall of the chorionic cavity is called the **chorion** and consists of three components: (1) extraembryonic somatic mesoderm, (2) cytotrophoblast, and (3) syncytiotrophoblast.

   B. Extraembryonic visceral mesoderm (splanchnopleuric mesoderm) covers the yolk sac.

IV. CLINICAL CORRELATIONS

   A. Human chorionic gonadotropin (HCG)

   1. HCG is a glycoprotein produced by the syncytiotrophoblast, which stimulates the production of progesterone by the corpus luteum (i.e., maintains corpus luteum function). This is clinically significant because **progesterone produced by the corpus luteum is essential for the maintenance of pregnancy until week 8.** The placenta then takes over the production of progesterone.

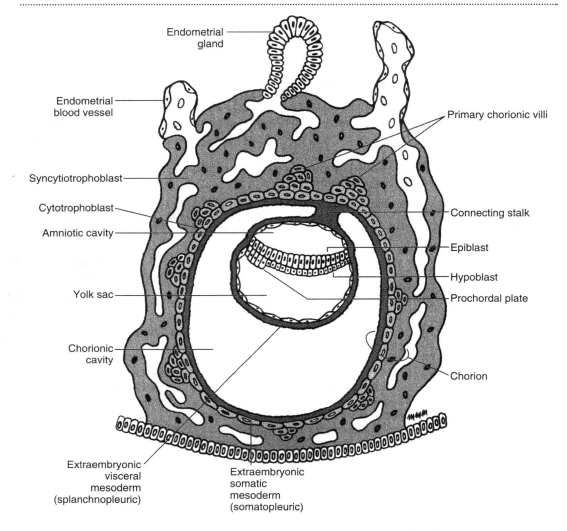

Figure 3-1.   Diagram of a day-14 blastocyst highlighting the formation of the bilaminar embryonic disk and the completion of implantation within the ondometrium.

        2. HCG can be assayed in maternal blood at day 8 or in maternal urine at day 10 and is the **basis of pregnancy testing.**

        3. HCG is detectable throughout a pregnancy. **Low HCG values** may predict a spontaneous abortion or indicate an ectopic pregnancy. **Elevated HCG values** may indicate a multiple pregnancy, hydatidiform mole, or gestational trophoblastic neoplasia.

    B. Hydatidiform mole. A blighted blastocyst leads to death of the embryo; this is followed by hyperplastic proliferation of the trophoblast, resulting in a vesicular or polycystic mass called a hydatidiform mole. Clinical signs diagnostic of a mole include preeclampsia during the first trimester, elevated HCG levels (>100,000 mIU/ml), and an enlarged uterus with bleeding. Follow-up visits are essential because 3%–5% of moles develop into gestational trophoblastic neoplasia.

C. **Gestational trophoblastic neoplasia (GTN; or choriocarcinoma).** GTN is a malignant tumor of the trophoblast that may occur after a normal or ectopic pregnancy, abortion, or hydatidiform mole. With a high degree of suspicion, elevated HCG levels are diagnostic. Nonmetastatic GTN (i.e., confined to the uterus) is the most common form of the neoplasia, and treatment is highly successful. However, the prognosis of metastatic GTN is poor if it spreads to the liver or brain.

D. **Oncofetal antigens** are cell surface antigens that normally appear only on embryonic cells; however, for unknown reasons, they re-express themselves in human malignant cells. Monoclonal antibodies directed against specific oncofetal antigens provide an avenue for cancer therapy.

   1. **Carcinoembryonic antigen (CEA)** is associated with colorectal carcinoma.

   2. **α-Fetoprotein** is associated with hepatoma and germ cell tumors.

E. **RU-486 (mifepristone)** will initiate menstruation when taken within 8–10 weeks of the previous menses. If implantation of a conceptus has occurred, the conceptus will be sloughed along with the endometrium. RU-486 which **blocks the progesterone receptor** is used in conjunction with prostaglandins and is 96% effective at terminating pregnancy.

4
Embryonic Period (Weeks 3–8)

I. INTRODUCTION. All major organ systems begin to develop during the embryonic period, causing a **craniocaudal and lateral body folding of the embryo.** By the end of the embryonic period (week 8), the embryo has a distinct human appearance. During the embryonic period, the basic segmentation of the human embryo in a craniocaudal direction is controlled by the **Hox (homeobox) complex** of genes. All Hox genes contain a 180-base pair sequence (**homeobox**) that encodes a 60 amino acid long region (**homeodomain**) that binds to DNA. All homeodomain proteins are gene regulatory proteins (i.e., they control transcription).

II. GASTRULATION (Figure 4-1) is a process that establishes the three primary germ layers of **ectoderm, mesoderm,** and **endoderm,** thereby forming **a trilaminar embryonic disk.** This process is first indicated by the formation of the **primitive streak** within the epiblast.

A. Ectoderm gives further rise to **neuroectoderm** and **neural crest cells.**

B. Endoderm remains intact.

C. Mesoderm gives further rise to **paraxial mesoderm** (somitomeres and 35 pairs of somites), **intermediate mesoderm,** and **lateral mesoderm.**

D. All adult cells and tissues can trace their embryologic origin back to the three primary germ layers (**Table 4-1**).

III. CLINICAL CORRELATIONS

A. Sacrococcygeal teratoma (Figure 4-2)

1. This tumor arises from **remnants of the primitive streak,** which normally degenerates and disappears.

2. A sacrococcygeal teratoma often contains various types of tissue (e.g., bone, nerve, hair) because it is derived from pluripotent cells of the primitive streak.

3. This tumor occurs more commonly in female infants.

4. The tumor usually becomes malignant during infancy and must be removed by 6 months of age.

B. Chordoma

1. This tumor arises from **remnants of the notochord.**

2. It may be found either intracranially or in the sacral region.

3. It occurs more commonly in men late in life (over age 50).

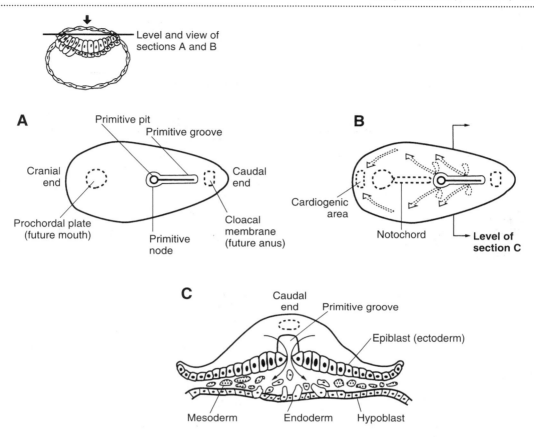

Figure 4-1. Gastrulation. The embryoblast in the upper left is provided for orientation. (A) Dorsal view of the epiblast. The primitive streak consists of the primitive groove, node, and pit. (B) *Arrows* show the migration of cells through the primitive streak. The notochord (i.e., mesoderm located between the primitive node and prochordal plate) induces the formation of the neural tube. The cardiogenic area is the future site of the heart. (C) Epiblast cells migrate to the primitive streak and insert themselves between the epiblast and hypoblast. Some epiblast cells displace the hypoblast to form endoderm; the remainder migrate cranially, laterally, and along the midline to form mesoderm. After gastrulation, the epiblast is called ectoderm.

   4. It may be either benign or malignant.

C. Caudal dysplasia (sirenomelia)

   1. The term "caudal dysplasia" refers to a **constellation of syndromes** ranging from minor lesions of the lower vertebrae to complete fusion of the lower limbs.

   2. This disorder is caused by abnormal gastrulation, in which the migration of mesoderm is disturbed.

   3. It can be associated with various cranial anomalies, such as:

Table 4-1

Summary of Germ Layer Derivatives

ECTODERM	Neuroectoderm

Epidermis, hair, nails, sweat and sebaceous glands
Utricle, semicircular ducts, vestibular ganglion of CN VIII
Saccule, cochlear duct, spiral ganglion of CN VIII
Olfactory placodes, CN I
Ameloblasts
Adenohypophysis
Lens of eye
Anterior epithelium of the cornea
Acinar cells of parotid gland
Acinar cells of mammary gland
Epithelial lining of:
    Lower anal canal
    Distal part of male urethra
    External auditory meatus
	All neurons within brain and spinal cord (CNS)
	Retina, iris, ciliary body, optic nerve (CNS), optic chiasm, optic tract, dilator and sphincter pupillae muscles
	Astrocytes, oligodendrocytes, ependymocytes, tanycytes, choroid plexus cells
	Neurohypophysis
	Pineal gland
	
	Neural crest:
	
	Ganglia (dorsal root, cranial, autonomic)
	Schwann cells
	Odontoblasts
	Pia and arachnoid
	Chromaffin cells (adrenal medulla)
	Parafollicular C cells of thyroid
	Melanocytes
	Aorticopulmonary septum
	Pharyngeal arch skeletal components
	Bones of neurocranium

MESODERM	**ENDODERM**

Muscle (smooth, cardiac, skeletal)
Extraocular muscles (preotic somites), ciliary muscle of eye, sclera, choroid, substantia propria of cornea, corneal endothelium
Muscles of tongue (occipital somites)
Pharyngeal arch muscles
Laryngeal cartilages
Connective tissue
Dermis of skin
Bone and cartilage
Dura mater
Endothelium of blood and lymph vessels
RBCs, WBCs, microglia, and Kupffer cells
Spleen
Kidney
Adrenal cortex
Testes and ovary
	Hepatocytes
	Principles and oxyphil of parathyroid
	Thyroid follicular cells
	Epithelial reticular cells of thymus
	Acinar and islet cells of pancreas
	Acinar cells of submandibular and sublingual glands
	Epithelial lining of:
	    GI tract
	    Trachea, bronchi, lungs
	    Biliary apparatus
	    Urinary bladder, female urethra, most of male urethra
	    Vagina
	    Auditory tube, middle ear cavity
	    Crypts of palatine tonsils

CN = cranial nerve; *CNS* = central nervous system; *GI* = gastrointestinal; *RBCs* = red blood cells; *WBCs* = white blood cells
(From Dudek RW, Fix JD: *Embryology,* 2nd ed. Baltimore, Williams & Wilkins, 1998, p. 36.)

    a. **VATER,** an acronym for vertebral defects, anal atresia, tracheoesophageal fistula, and renal defects
    b. **VACTERL,** which is similar to VATER but also includes cardiovascular defects and upper limb defects

  D. Missed menstrual period
    1. A missed period is usually **the first indication of pregnancy.** Week 3 of embryonic

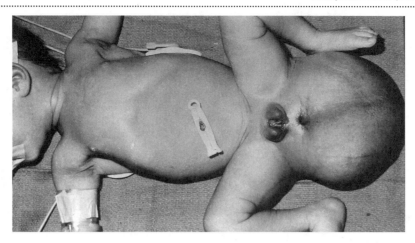

Figure 4-2.   Infant with a sacrococcygeal teratoma. (From Sadler TW: *Langman's Medical Embryology,* 7th ed. Baltimore, Williams & Wilkins, 1995, p 62.)

    development coincides with the first missed menstrual period. (Note that at this time the embryo has already undergone 2 weeks of development.)

2. It is crucial that the woman becomes aware of a pregnancy as soon as possible because the embryonic period is a **period of high susceptibility to teratogens.**

5

Placenta, Amniotic Fluid, and Umbilical Cord

I. PLACENTA (Figure 5-1)

A. Components

1. The **maternal component** of the placenta consists of a portion of the endometrium called the **decidua basalis.**

2. The **fetal component** of the placenta consists of tertiary chorionic villi, which are collectively called the **villous chorion.**

B. Afterbirth appearance of the placenta

1. The **maternal surface** of the placenta is characterized by **15–20 cotyledons** that impart a cobblestone appearance. The surface is dark red and oozes blood after birth owing to torn maternal blood vessels.

2. The **fetal surface** of the placenta is characterized by the **chorionic blood vessels.** It appears smooth and shiny because the amnion covers this surface.

C. Clinical correlations

1. **Velamentous placenta** occurs when the umbilical vessels abnormally travel through the amniochorionic membrane before reaching the placenta proper. If the umbilical vessels cross the internal os, a serious condition called **vasa previa** exists. In vasa previa, if one of the **umbilical vessels ruptures** during pregnancy, labor, or delivery, the fetus will bleed to death.

2. **Placenta previa** occurs when the placenta attaches in the lower part of the uterus, **covering the internal os.** (The placenta normally implants in the posterior superior wall of the uterus.) **Uterine vessels rupture** during the later part of pregnancy as the uterus begins to gradually dilate. The mother may bleed to death, and the fetus will also be placed in jeopardy because of the compromised blood supply.

a. Placenta previa is clinically associated with repeated **episodes of bright red vaginal bleeding.**

b. Because the placenta blocks the cervical opening, delivery is usually accomplished by **cesarean section.**

3. **Placenta as an allograft.** The fetal component of the placenta inherits both paternal and maternal genes and, therefore, may be considered as an allograft with respect to the mother. However, the placenta is not rejected in most cases. The two factors responsible for the lack of rejection are:

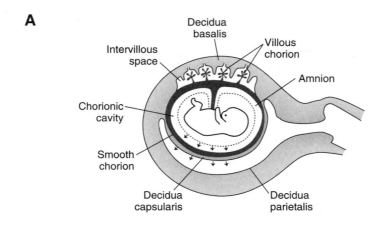

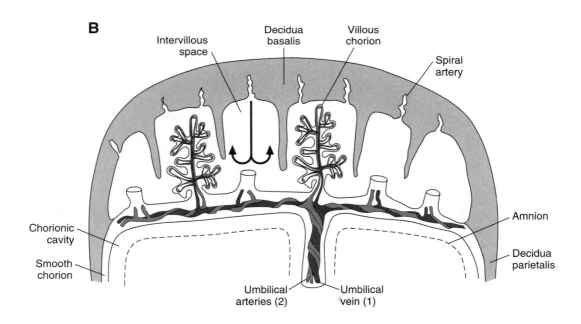

Figure 5-1. (A) Relationship of the fetus, uterus, and placenta in the early fetal period. The *outer arrows* indicate that as the fetus grows within the uterine wall the decidua capsularis expands and fuses with the decidua parietalis, thereby obliterating the uterine cavity. The *inner arrows* indicate that as the fetus grows, the amnion expands toward the smooth chorion, thus obliterating the chorionic cavity. (B) Diagram of the placenta. This diagram of the placenta is oriented in the same direction as (A) for comparison. Note the relationship of the villous chorion (fetal component) to the decidua basalis (maternal component). Maternal blood enters the intervillous space (*curved arrow*) via the spiral arteries and bathes the villi in maternal blood. The villi contain fetal capillaries and thus maternal and fetal blood exchange occurs.

    a. Syncytiotrophoblast cells lining the villous chorion **lack major histocompatibility complex (MHC) antigens** and thus do not evoke an immune response.

    b. Decidual cells within the endometrial stroma secrete **prostaglandin E_2,** which inhibits T lymphocyte activation.

4. Preeclampsia and eclampsia. Preeclampsia refers to the sudden development of **maternal hypertension, edema, and proteinuria** usually after week 32 of gestation. Eclampsia includes the additional symptom of **convulsions.**

    a. Risk factors include nulliparity, diabetes, hypertension, renal disease, twin gestation, or hydatidiform mole (produces first trimester preeclampsia).

    b. The cause is abnormal placentation producing a mechanical or functional obstruction of the spiral arteries of the uterus.

    c. Treatment consists in delivery of the baby as soon as possible.

5. Twinning (Figure 5-2)

    a. Dizygotic (fraternal) twins develop from two zygotes. The fetuses have **two placentas, two chorions,** and **two amniotic sacs.**

    b. Monozygotic (identical) twins develop from one zygote. In **65% of cases,** the fetuses have one placenta, one chorion, and two amniotic sacs. In the remaining **35% of cases,** the fetuses have two placentas (separate or fused), two chorions, and two amniotic sacs.

II. PLACENTAL MEMBRANE

A. Layers

1. In early pregnancy, the placental membrane consists of the **syncytiotrophoblast, cytotrophoblast (Langerhans cells), connective tissue,** and **endothelium of the fetal capillaries.** Hofbauer cells are found in the connective tissue and are most likely macrophages.

2. In late pregnancy, the cytotrophoblast degenerates and the connective tissue is displaced by the growth of fetal capillaries, leaving the **syncytiotrophoblast** and the **fetal capillary endothelium.**

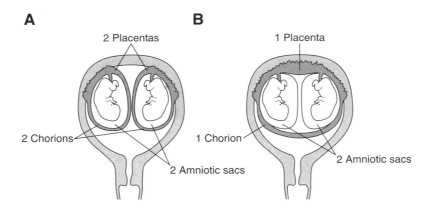

Figure 5-2. Arrangement of the placenta, chorion, and amniotic sac of (A) dizygotic twins and 35% of monozygotic twins and (B) 65% of monozygotic twins. In general, dizygotic twins can be distinguished from monozygotic twins by an inspection of the afterbirth. However, please note that in approximately 35% of cases the determination will be in error.

B. Function. The placental membrane **separates maternal blood from fetal blood.** Some substances (both beneficial and harmful to the fetus) cross the placental membrane freely, whereas it is impermeable to others **(Table 5-1).**

C. Clinical correlation. Erythroblastosis fetalis occurs when **Rh-positive fetal red blood cells** (RBCs) cross the placental membrane into the maternal circulation of an **Rh-negative mother.** The mother forms anti-Rh antibodies that cross the placental membrane and destroy fetal RBCs, which leads to:

1. The release of large amounts of **bilirubin** (a breakdown product of hemoglobin) that may cause brain damage

2. Severe hemolytic disease whereby the fetus is severely anemic and demonstrates

Table 5-1
Substances That Cross or Do Not Cross the Placental Membrane

BENEFICIAL SUBSTANCES THAT CROSS THE PLACENTAL MEMBRANE

- Oxygen, carbon dioxide
- Glucose, amino acids, free fatty acids, vitamins
- Water, sodium, potassium, chloride, calcium, phosphate
- Urea, uric acid, bilirubin
- Fetal and maternal RBCs
- Maternal serum proteins, α-fetoprotein
- Steroid hormones (unconjugated)
- IgG (confers passive immunity)

HARMFUL SUBSTANCES THAT CROSS THE PLACENTAL MEMBRANE*

- Viruses—e.g., rubella, cytomegalovirus, herpes simplex type 2, varicella zoster, Coxsackie, variola, measles, poliomyelitis

- Category X Drugs (absolute contraindication in pregnancy)—e.g., thalidomide, aminopterin, methotrexate, busulfan (Myleran), chlorambucil (Leukeran), cyclophosphamide (Cytoxan), phenytoin (Dilantin), triazolam (Halcion), estazolam (ProSom), warfarin (Coumadin), isotretinoin (Accutane), clomiphene (Clomid), diethylstilbestrol (DES), ethisterone, norethisterone, megestrol (Megace), oral contraceptives (Ovcon, Levlen, Norinyl), nicotine, alcohol

- Category D Drugs (definite evidence of risk to fetus)—e.g., tetracycline (Achromycin), doxycycline (Vibramycin), streptomycin, Amikacin, tobramycin (Nebcin), phenobarbital (Donnatal), pentobarbital (Nembutal), valproic acid (Depakene), diazepam (Valium), chlordiazepoxide (Librium), alprazolam (Xanax), lorazepam (Ativan), lithium, chlorothiazide (Diuril)

- Carbon monoxide
- Organic mercury, lead, polychlorinated biphenyls (PCBs), potassium iodide,
- Cocaine, heroin
- *Toxoplasma gondii, Treponema palladium*
- Rubella virus vaccine
- Anti-Rh antibodies

SUBSTANCES THAT DO NOT CROSS THE PLACENTAL MEMBRANE

- Maternally-derived cholesterol, triglycerides, and phospholipids
- Protein hormones (e.g., insulin)
- Drugs (e.g., succinylcholine, curare, heparin, methyldopa, drugs similar to amino acids)
- IgA, IgD, IgE, IgM
- Bacteria

*See Chapter 26

total body edema (**hydrops fetalis**), which may lead to death. In these cases, an intrauterine transfusion is indicated.

III. AMNIOTIC FLUID is basically water that contains carbohydrates, lipids, proteins (e.g., hormones, enzymes, α-fetoprotein), desquamated fetal cells, and fetal urine.

A. **Production.** Amniotic fluid is produced by **dialysis of maternal and fetal blood** through blood vessels in the placenta and by **excretion of fetal urine** into the amniotic sac.

B. **Resorption.** After being swallowed by the fetus, the amniotic fluid is removed by the placenta and passed into the maternal blood.

C. Clinical correlations

1. Oligohydramnios occurs when there is a **low amount of amniotic fluid** (< 400 ml in late pregnancy). Oligohydramnios may be associated with the inability of the fetus to excrete urine into the amniotic sac due to **renal agenesis.** This results in many fetal deformities (**Potter's syndrome**) and **hypoplastic lungs** due to increased pressure on the fetal thorax.

2. **Polyhydramnios** occurs when the **level of amniotic fluid is high** (>2000 ml in late pregnancy). Polyhydramnios may be associated with the inability of the fetus to swallow due to **anencephaly** or **esophageal atresia.** Polyhydramnios is commonly associated with **maternal diabetes.**

3. **α-Fetoprotein (AFP)** is "fetal albumin," which is produced by fetal hepatocytes. It is routinely assayed in amniotic fluid and maternal serum between **weeks 14 and 18** of gestation. AFP levels change with gestational age so that proper interpretation of AFP levels depends on an accurate gestational age.
   a. **Elevated AFP levels** are associated with **neural tube defects** (e.g., **spina bifida or anencephaly**), **omphalocele** (allows fetal serum to leak into the amniotic fluid), **esophageal and duodenal atresia** (which interfere with fetal swallowing).
   b. **Reduced AFP levels** are associated with **Down syndrome.**

4. **Premature rupture of the amniochorionic membrane** is the most common cause of premature labor and oligohydramnios. (Rupture of the amniochorionic membrane is commonly referred to as "breaking of the water bag.")

5. **Amniotic band syndrome** occurs when bands of amniotic membrane encircle and constrict parts of the fetus causing **limb amputations** and **craniofacial anomalies.**

IV. UMBILICAL CORD. The definitive umbilical cord contains the right and left umbilical arteries, left umbilical vein, and mucous connective tissue.

A. The **umbilical arteries** carry **deoxygenated blood** from the fetus to the placenta.

B. The **left umbilical vein** carries **oxygenated blood** from the placenta to the fetus.

C. Clinical correlations

1. The presence of **only one umbilical artery** within the umbilical cord is an abnormal finding that suggests **cardiovascular abnormalities.** (Normally, two umbilical arteries are present.)

2. **Physical inspection of the umbilicus** in a newborn infant may reveal:
   a. A light gray shining sac indicating an **omphalocele** (see Chapter 7).
   b. Fecal (meconium) discharge indicating a **vitelline fistula** (see Chapter 7).
   c. Urine discharge indicating a **urachal fistula** (see Chapter 8).

V. VASCULOGENESIS (de novo Blood Vessel Formation)

    A. Mesoderm differentiates into **angioblasts** that form **angiogenic cell clusters.**

    B. Angioblasts around the periphery of the angiogenic cell clusters give rise to the **endothelium** of blood vessels.

    C. Vasculogenesis occurs initially in **extraembryonic visceral mesoderm around the yolk sac** on day 17 and later in mesoderm within the fetus.

VI. HEMATOPOIESIS (Blood Cell Formation; Figure 5-3)

    A. Mesoderm differentiates into **angioblasts,** which form **angiogenic cell clusters.**

    B. Angioblasts within the center of angiogenic cell clusters give rise to primitive **blood cells.**

    C. Hematopoiesis occurs initially in **extraembryonic visceral mesoderm around the yolk sac** during week 3.

    D. Beginning in week 5, hematopoiesis is taken over by a sequence of embryonic organs: **liver, spleen, thymus, and bone marrow.**

    E. Several **types of hemoglobin** are produced during hematopoiesis.

        1. During the period of yolk sac hematopoiesis, the earliest **embryonic form** of hemoglobin, called **hemoglobin $\delta_2\epsilon_2$,** is synthesized.

        2. During the period of liver hematopoiesis, the **fetal form** of hemoglobin, called **hemoglobin $\alpha_2\gamma_2$,** is synthesized. Hemoglobin $\alpha_2\gamma_2$ is the predominant form of hemoglobin during pregnancy because it has a higher affinity for oxygen than does the adult form of hemoglobin (hemoglobin $\alpha_2\beta_2$) and thus "pulls" oxygen from the maternal blood into fetal blood.

        3. During the period of bone marrow hematopoiesis (approximately week 30), the **adult form** of hemoglobin, called **hemoglobin $\alpha_2\beta_2$,** is synthesized and gradually replaces hemoglobin $\alpha_2\gamma_2$.

    F. **Clinical correlation. Thalassemia syndromes** constitute a heterogeneous group of genetic defects characterized by the lack of or decreased synthesis of either the α-globin chain (**α-thalassemia**) or β-globin chain (**β-thalassemia**) of hemoglobin $\alpha_2\beta_2$.

        1. **Hydrops fetalis** is the most severe form of α-thalassemia. It causes severe pallor,

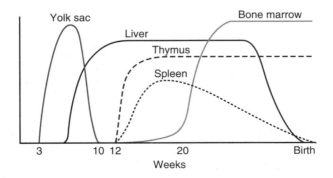

Figure 5-3. Diagram showing the contribution of various organs to hematopoiesis during embryonic and fetal development.

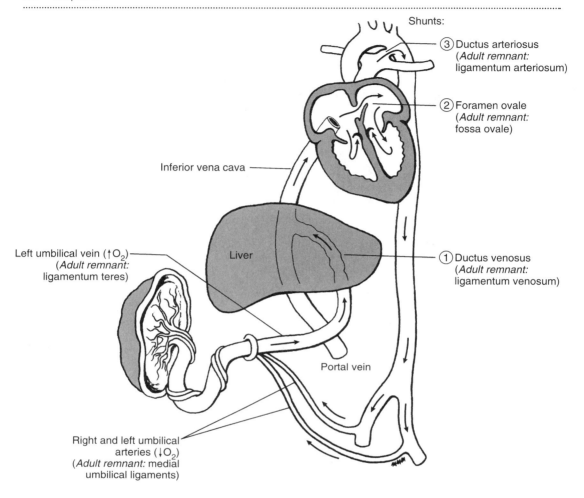

Shunts:

③ Ductus arteriosus
(*Adult remnant:*
ligamentum arteriosum)

② Foramen ovale
(*Adult remnant:*
fossa ovale)

Inferior vena cava

Left umbilical vein ($\uparrow O_2$)
(*Adult remnant:*
ligamentum teres)

Liver

① Ductus venosus
(*Adult remnant:*
ligamentum venosum)

Portal vein

Right and left umbilical
arteries ($\downarrow O_2$)
(*Adult remnant:* medial
umbilical ligaments)

Figure 5-4.   Fetal circulation. Note the three shunts and the changes that occur after birth (remnants).

Table 5-2

Remnants Created by Closure of Fetal Circulatory Structures

Fetal Structure	Adult Remnant
Right and left umbilical arteries	Medial umbilical ligaments
Left umbilical vein	Ligamentum teres
Ductus venosus	Ligamentum venosum
Foramen ovale	Fossa ovale
Ductus arteriosus	Ligamentum arteriosum

generalized edema, and massive hepatosplenomegaly and leads invariably to intrauterine fetal death.

2. **β-Thalassemia major** is the most severe form of β-thalassemia, It causes a severe, transfusion-dependent anemia. It is most common in Mediterranean countries and in parts of Africa and Southeast Asia.

VII. **FETAL CIRCULATION** involves three shunts: (1) **ductus venosus,** (2) **foramen ovale,** and (3) **ductus arteriosus (Figure 5-4).** Several changes occur in the neonatal circulation when **right atrial pressure decreases** owing to occlusion of placental circulation and when **left atrial pressure increases** due to increased pulmonary venous return from the lungs. **Table 5-2** summarizes the remnants that result from closure of the fetal structures.

6

Cardiovascular System

I. DEVELOPMENT OF THE PRIMITIVE HEART TUBE. A pair of **endocardial heart tubes** (mesodermal in origin) form within the cardiogenic region.

A. As lateral folding occurs, the endocardial heart tubes fuse to form the **primitive heart tube,** which develops into the **endocardium.**

B. Mesoderm surrounding the primitive heart tube develops into the **myocardium** and **epicardium.**

C. The primitive heart tube forms **five dilatations: truncus arteriosus, bulbus cordis, primitive ventricle, primitive atrium, and sinus venosus.** The fate of each dilatation is described in **Figure 6-1.**

II. DEVELOPMENT OF HEART SEPTAE. The primitive heart tube is a tube with a single lumen. This single lumen is partitioned into four definitive chambers by the formation of four septae: **aorticopulmonary (AP), atrioventricular (AV), atrial,** and **interventricular (IV).** Many congenital heart defects can be traced back to the abnormal formation of these septae.

A. **Aorticopulmonary (AP) septum (Figure 6-2).** The AP septum divides the truncus arteriosus into the **aorta** and **pulmonary trunk.**

1. **Formation.** Neural crest cells migrate into the **truncal** and **bulbar ridges,** which grow in a spiral fashion and fuse to form the AP septum.

2. Clinical correlations
a. **Persistent truncus arteriosus** is caused by abnormal neural crest cell migration such that there is only partial development of the AP septum. This results in a condition in which only one large vessel leaves the heart, and it receives blood from both the right and left ventricles. The resultant **right-to-left shunting** of blood leads to **cyanosis.**
b. **D-Transposition of the great vessels (complete)** is caused by abnormal neural crest cell migration such that there is nonspiral development of the AP septum. This results in a condition in which the aorta arises abnormally from the right ventricle and the pulmonary trunk arises abnormally from the left ventricle. The resultant **right-to-left shunting** of blood leads to **cyanosis.**
c. **Tetralogy of Fallot** is caused by abnormal neural crest cell migration such that there is skewed development of the AP septum. This results in a condition classically characterized by: **pulmonary stenosis, overriding aorta, IV septal defect,** and **right ventricular hypertrophy.** The resultant **right-to-left shunting** of blood leads to **cyanosis.**

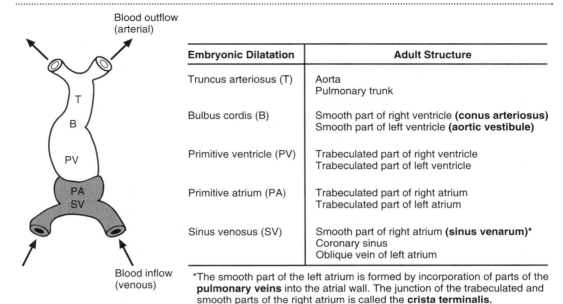

Blood outflow
(arterial)

Blood inflow
(venous)

Embryonic Dilatation	Adult Structure
Truncus arteriosus (T)	Aorta Pulmonary trunk
Bulbus cordis (B)	Smooth part of right ventricle **(conus arteriosus)** Smooth part of left ventricle **(aortic vestibule)**
Primitive ventricle (PV)	Trabeculated part of right ventricle Trabeculated part of left ventricle
Primitive atrium (PA)	Trabeculated part of right atrium Trabeculated part of left atrium
Sinus venosus (SV)	Smooth part of right atrium **(sinus venarum)*** Coronary sinus Oblique vein of left atrium

*The smooth part of the left atrium is formed by incorporation of parts of the **pulmonary veins** into the atrial wall. The junction of the trabeculated and smooth parts of the right atrium is called the **crista terminalis.**

Figure 6-1.   The five embryonic dilatations of the primitive heart tube, and the adult structures derived from them.

B.   Atrioventricular (AV) septum (Figure 6-3). The AV septum divides the AV canal into the **right AV canal** and **left AV canal.**

   1.   Formation. The **dorsal** and **ventral AV cushions** fuse to form the AV septum.

   2.   Clinical correlations
      a.   Univentricular heart is caused by an extremely skewed development of the AV septum to the right. This results in a condition in which one ventricle receives both the tricuspid and mitral valves.
      b.   Tricuspid atresia is caused by an insufficient amount of AV cushion tissue available for the formation of the tricuspid valve. This results in a condition in which there is complete agenesis of the tricuspid valve so that no communication exists between the right atrium and right ventricle. Tricuspid atresia is characterized by: a **patent foramen ovale, IV septal defect, overdeveloped left ventricle,** and **underdeveloped right ventricle.**

C.   Atrial septum (Figure 6-4). The atrial septum divides the primitive atrium into the **right** and **left atria.**

   1.   Formation
      a.   The septum primum grows toward the AV septum.
      b.   The foramen primum is located between the edge of septum primum and the AV septum; it is obliterated when the septum primum fuses with the AV septum.
      c.   The foramen secundum forms in the center of the septum primum.
      d.   The septum secundum forms to the right of the septum primum and fuses (after birth) with the septum primum to form the atrial septum.
      e.   The foramen ovale is the opening between the upper and lower parts of the septum secundum. During fetal life, blood is shunted from the right atrium to the left atrium via the foramen ovale. Closure of the foramen ovale normally

A. Formation of the Aorticopulmonary (AP) Septum

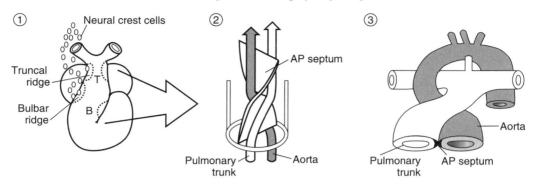

B. AP Septal Defects

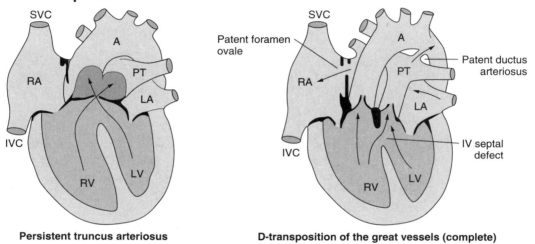

Persistent truncus arteriosus

D-transposition of the great vessels (complete)

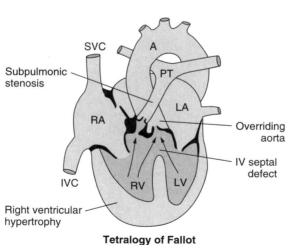

Tetralogy of Fallot

Figure 6-2. (*A*) Formation of the aorticopulmonary (AP) septum. ①Partitioning of the truncus arteriosus and bulbus cordis, involving neural crest cell migration. ②The AP septum develops in a spiral fashion. ③The spiral AP septum accounts for the adult gross anatomic relationship between the aorta (*shaded*) and the pulmonary trunk (*unshaded*). (*B*) AP septal defects: persistent truncus arteriosus, D-transposition of the great vessels (complete), and tetralogy of Fallot.

A. Formation of the Atrioventricular (AV) Septum

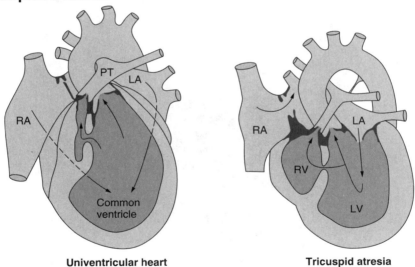

① Ventral AV cushion

A

Dorsal AV cushion

V

Single AV canal

② Level of section ③

A

AV septum

V

③ AV septum

Right AV canal   Left AV canal

B. AV Septal Defects

PT   LA

RA

Common ventricle

Univentricular heart

RA   LA

RV

LV

Tricuspid atresia

Figure 6-3. (A) Formation of the atrioventricular (AV) septum: The partitioning of the AV canal. (B) AV septal defects: univentricular heart and tricuspid atresia. A = atrium; AV = atrioventricular; V = ventricle; RA = right atrium; RV = right ventricle; LA = left atrium; LV = left ventricle.

occur soon after birth and is facilitated by the **increased left atrial pressure** that results from changes in pulmonary circulation.

    2. Clinical correlations. Heart defects involving the atrial septum are called atrial septal defects **(ASDs).**

        a. Foramen secundum defect is caused by excessive resorption of the septum primum, septum secundum, or both. This results in an opening between the right and left atria **(patent foramen ovale).** If the ASD is small, clinical symptoms may be delayed as late as age 30. This is the most common clinically significant ASD.

A. Formation of the Atrial Septum

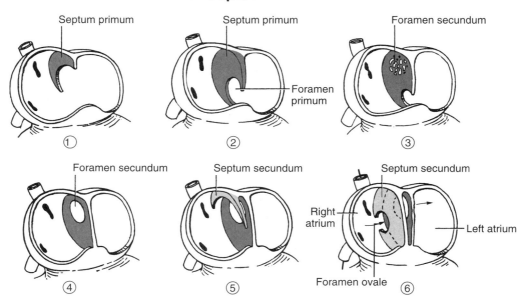

B. Atrial Septum Defect (ASD)

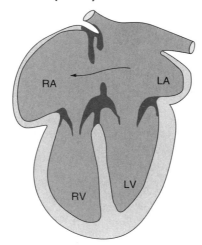

Foramen secundum defect

Figure 6-4. (A) Formation of the atrial septum. The *arrows* in ⑥ indicate the direction of blood flow across the fully developed septum, from the right atrium to the left atrium. (B) An atrial septal defect: foramen secundum defect. The *arrow* indicates the abnormal flow of blood through the defect.

    b. **Premature closure of foramen ovale** is the closure of the foramen ovale during prenatal life. This results in hypertrophy of the right side of the heart and underdevelopment of the left side.

  D. **Interventricular (IV) septum (Figure 6-5).** The IV septum divides the primitive ventricle into the **right** and **left ventricles.**

A. Formation of the Interventricular (IV) Septum

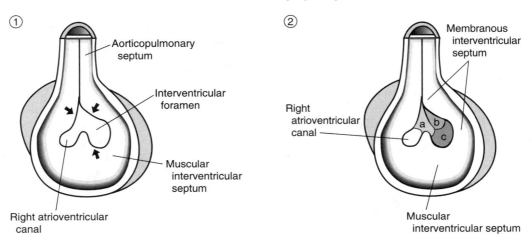

B. IV Septal Defect

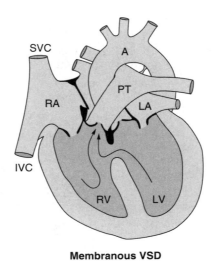

Membranous VSD

Figure 6-5. (A) Formation of the interventricular (IV) septum: partitioning of the primitive ventricle. *Shaded portions* (a, b, c) in ② indicate the three components of the membranous IV septum. *a* = right bulbar ridge; *b* = left bulbar ridge; *c* = AV cushions. (B) an IV septal defect: Membranous VSD. *Arrows* indicate the direction of blood flow. A = aorta; *IVC* = inferior vena cava; *LA* = left atrium; *LV* = left ventricle; *PT* = pulmonary trunk; *RA* = right atrium; *RV* = right ventricle; *SVC* = superior vena cava.

1. **Formation**
   a. The **muscular IV septum** develops in the floor of the ventricle; it grows toward the AV cushions but stops short leaving the **IV foramen.**
   b. The **membranous IV septum** forms by the fusion of three components: the **right bulbar ridge, left bulbar ridge,** and **AV cushions.** This fusion closes the IV foramen.

2. **Clinical correlation. A membranous ventricular septal defect (VSD)** is caused by incomplete fusion of the right bulbar ridge, left bulbar ridge, and AV cushions. This results in a condition in which an opening between the right and left ventricles allows **left-to-right shunting** of blood through the IV foramen. Patients with left-to-right shunting complain of **excessive fatigue upon exertion.**
   a. Initially, a membranous VSD is associated with left-to-right shunting of blood, increased pulmonary blood flow, and pulmonary hypertension.
   b. Later, the pulmonary hypertension causes marked proliferation of the tunica intima and tunica media of pulmonary muscular arteries and arterioles, thus narrowing their lumen.
   c. Ultimately, pulmonary resistance becomes higher than systemic resistance and causes **right-to-left shunting** of blood and **cyanosis.** At this stage, the condition is called the **Eisenmenger complex.**

Table 6-1
Development of the Arterial System

Embryonic Structure	Adult Structure
Aortic arches	
1	*
2	*
3	Common carotid arteries Internal carotid arteries (proximal part)
4	Right subclavian artery (proximal part) Part of the aortic arch
5	Regresses in the human
6	Pulmonary arteries (proximal part)
	Ductus arteriosus†
Dorsal aorta	
Posterolateral branches	Arteries to upper and lower extremity Intercostal, lumbar, and lateral sacral arteries
Lateral branches	Renal, suprarenal, and gonadal arteries
Ventral branches Vitelline arteries	Celiac, superior mesenteric, and inferior mesenteric arteries
Umbilical arteries	Part of internal iliac arteries, superior vesical arteries Medial umbilical ligaments

*Minimal contribution in the adult
†Early in development, the recurrent laryngeal nerves hook around aortic arch 6. On the right side, the distal part of aortic arch 6 regresses, and the right recurrent laryngeal nerve moves up to hook around the right subclavian artery. On the left side, aortic arch 6 persists as the ductus arteriosus (or ligamentum arteriosus in the adult); the left recurrent laryngeal nerve remains hooked around the ductus arteriosus.

Table 6-2
Development of Venous System

Embryonic Structure	Adult Structure
Vitelline veins	
Right and left	Hepatic veins and sinusoids, ductus venosus, part of the IVC, portal vein, superior mesenteric vein, inferior mesenteric vein, and splenic vein
Umbilical veins	
Right	Regresses early in development
Left	Ligamentum teres
Cardinal veins	Internal jugular veins, SVC, part of the IVC, common iliac veins, renal veins, gonadal veins, intercostal veins, hemiazygos vein, and azygos vein

IVC = inferior vena cava; *SVC* = superior vena cava.

III. DEVELOPMENT OF THE ARTERIAL SYSTEM (Table 6-1)

- **A. Formation.** The arterial system develops from the **aortic arches** (contributes to arteries in the head and neck region) and the **dorsal aorta** (which contributes to arteries in the rest of the body). The dorsal aorta sprouts posterolateral, lateral, and ventral branches (i.e., vitelline and umbilical arteries).

- **B. Clinical correlations**

  - **1.** **Postductal coarctation of the aorta** occurs when the aorta is abnormally constricted just distal to the ductus arteriosus and left subclavian artery.
    - **a.** This condition is clinically associated with **increased blood pressure in the upper extremities, lack of a femoral pulse, and a high risk of both cerebral hemorrhage and bacterial endocarditis.**
    - **b.** Collateral circulation around the constriction involves the internal thoracic, intercostal, superior epigastric, inferior epigastric, and external iliac arteries. Dilatation of the intercostal arteries causes erosion of the lower border of the ribs (called "**rib notching**"), which can be seen on a radiograph.

  - **2.** **Patent ductus arteriosus (PDA)** occurs when the ductus arteriosus, a connection between the left pulmonary artery and the arch of the aorta, fails to close. Normally, the ductus arteriosus closes within a few hours after birth via smooth muscle contraction to form the ligamentum arteriosum.
    - **a.** PDA causes a left-to-right shunting of blood from the aorta back into the pulmonary circulation.
    - **b.** PDA is very common in **premature infants** and in infants born to mothers who contracted the **rubella virus** during the course of their pregnancy.
    - **c.** Prostaglandin E, intrauterine asphyxia, and neonatal asphyxia sustain the patency of the ductus arteriosus.
    - **d.** Prostaglandin inhibitors (e.g., indomethacin), acetylcholine, histamine, and catecholamines promote closure of the ductus arteriosus.

IV. DEVELOPMENT OF THE VENOUS SYSTEM (Table 6-2). The venous system develops from the **vitelline, umbilical,** and **cardinal veins** that empty into the sinus venosus. These veins undergo remodeling owing to a redirection of venous blood from the left side of the body to the right side in order to empty into the right atrium.

7

Digestive System

I. PRIMITIVE GUT TUBE. The primitive gut tube is divided into the **foregut, midgut,** and **hindgut (Figure 7-1).**

A. Formation. The primitive gut tube is formed by the incorporation of a portion of the yolk sac into the embryo during craniocaudal and lateral folding.

B. Histology. The epithelial lining and glands of the mucosa are derived from **endoderm,** whereas the lamina propria, muscularis mucosae, submucosa, muscularis externa, and adventitia/serosa are derived from **mesoderm.** The epithelial lining of the gut tube proliferates rapidly and obliterates the lumen. Later, **recanalization** occurs.

II. FOREGUT DERIVATIVES are supplied by the **celiac artery.**

A. Esophagus

1. Formation. The **tracheoesophageal septum** divides the foregut into the esophagus and trachea.

2. Clinical correlation: Esophageal atresia occurs when the esophagus ends as a blind tube owing to a malformation of the tracheoesophageal septum. It is associated with polyhydramnios and a tracheoesophageal fistula (see Chapter 10).

B. Stomach

1. Formation. The primitive stomach develops from a fusiform dilatation that forms in the foregut during week 4. The stomach rotates 90 degrees clockwise during its formation, causing the formation of the lesser peritoneal sac.

2. Clinical correlation. Hypertrophic pyloric stenosis occurs when the muscularis externa hypertrophies, narrowing the pyloric lumen. This condition is associated with projectile nonbilious vomiting and a small, palpable mass at the right costal margin.

C. Liver

1. Formation. The hepatic diverticulum sends **hepatic cell cords** into the surrounding mesoderm called the **septum transversum.** As the liver bulges into the abdominal cavity, the septum transversum is stretched to form the **ventral mesentery.** The septum transversum also plays a role in the formation of the **diaphragm,** which explains the close adult anatomic relationship of the liver and diaphragm.

2. Clinical correlation. Congenital malformations of the liver are rare.

D. Gallbladder and bile ducts

1. Formation. The connection between the hepatic diverticulum and foregut nar-

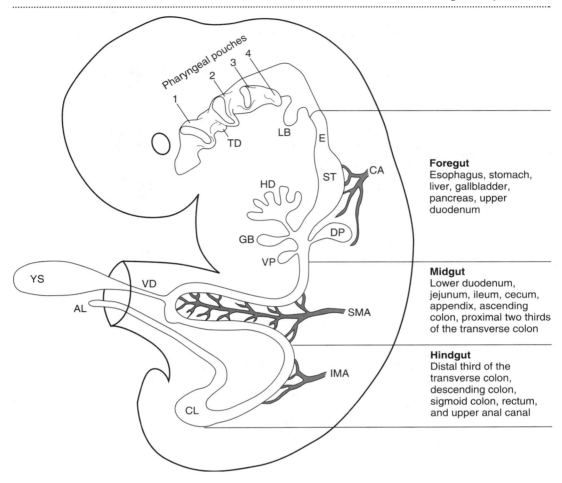

Foregut
Esophagus, stomach,
liver, gallbladder,
pancreas, upper
duodenum

Midgut
Lower duodenum,
jejunum, ileum, cecum,
appendix, ascending
colon, proximal two thirds
of the transverse colon

Hindgut
Distal third of the
transverse colon,
descending colon,
sigmoid colon, rectum,
and upper anal canal

Figure 7-1. Development of gastrointestinal tract showing the foregut, midgut, and hindgut along with the adult derivatives. The entire length of the endodermal gut tube is shown from the mouth to the anus. The fate of the lung bud (LB) is covered in Chapter 10. The fate of the pharyngeal pouches (1, 2, 3, 4) and the thyroid diverticulum (TD) are covered in Chapter 11. E = esophagus; ST = stomach; HD = hepatic diverticulum; GB = gallbladder; VP = ventral pancreatic bud; DP = dorsal pancreatic bud; CA = celiac artery; YS = yolk sac; VD = vitelline duct; AL = allantois; SMA = superior mesenteric artery; CL = cloaca; IMA = inferior mesenteric artery.

rows to form the bile duct. Later, an outgrowth from the bile duct gives rise to the gallbladder and cystic duct.

   2. Clinical correlation. Extrahepatic biliary atresia occurs when incomplete re-canalization leads to occlusion of the biliary ducts. This condition is associated with jaundice soon after birth, pale stool, and dark urine.

E. Pancreas

   1. Formation. The **ventral pancreatic bud** forms the uncinate process and part of the head of the pancreas. The **dorsal pancreatic bud** forms the remaining part of the head, body, and tail of the pancreas. Acinar cells, duct epithelium, and islet cells are derived from endoderm.

   2. Clinical correlations

   a. **Annular pancreas** occurs when the ventral and dorsal pancreatic buds form a ring around the duodenum, thus causing an obstruction of the duodenum.

   b. **Macrosomia (increased birthweight)** occurs when fetal islets are exposed to high glucose levels such as those present in a pregnancy involving an uncontrolled diabetic woman. Glucose freely crosses the placenta and stimulates fetal insulin secretion, which causes increased fat and glycogen deposition in fetal tissues.

F. **Upper duodenum.** The upper duodenum develops from the **caudal portion of the foregut.** The junction of the foregut and midgut is just **distal to the opening of the common bile duct.**

III. MIDGUT DERIVATIVES are supplied by the **superior mesenteric artery.**

A. Lower duodenum

   1. **Formation.** The lower duodenum develops from the **cranial portion of the midgut.**

   2. **Clinical correlation. Duodenal atresia** occurs when the lumen of the duodenum is occluded owing to failed recanalization. This condition is associated with polyhydramnios, bile-containing vomitus, and distended stomach.

B. **Jejunum, ileum, cecum, appendix, ascending colon, and proximal two thirds of the transverse colon**

   1. **Formation.** At week 6, the **midgut loop** herniates through the primitive umbilical ring and causes a **physiologic umbilical herniation.** At week 11, the midgut loop rotates **270 degrees counterclockwise** around the **superior mesenteric artery** as it returns to the abdominal cavity, thus reducing the physiologic umbilical herniation.

   2. Clinical correlations

   a. **Omphalocele** occurs when the midgut loop fails to return to the abdominal cavity. In the newborn, a light gray shiny sac protruding from the base of the umbilical cord is apparent **(Figure 7-2A).**

   b. **Ileal (Meckel's) diverticulum** occurs when a remnant of the vitelline duct persists, thus forming a blind pouch on the antimesenteric border of the ileum. This condition is often asymptomatic but occasionally becomes inflamed or contains ectopic gastric, pancreatic, or endometrial tissue, which may produce ulceration.

   c. **Vitelline fistula** occurs when the vitelline duct persists, thus forming a direct connection between the intestinal lumen and the outside of the body at the umbilicus. This condition is associated with fecal (meconium) discharge from the umbilicus.

   d. **Malrotation of the midgut** occurs when the midgut undergoes only partial rotation and results in the abnormal position of abdominal viscera. This condition may be associated with **volvulus** (twisting of intestines), which can compromise blood flow and result in gangrene.

   e. **Intestinal atresia or stenosis** occurs as a result of failed recanalization.

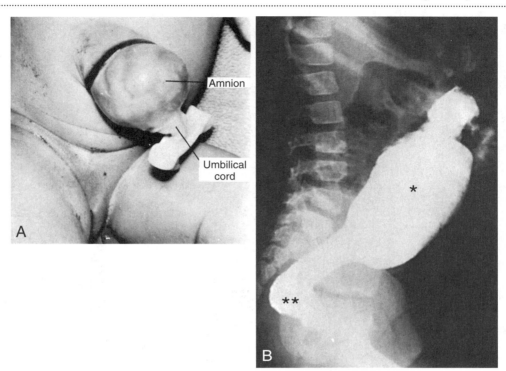

Figure 7-2. (A) Photograph of a newborn infant with an omphalocele that is covered by amnion and contains loops of intestine. (B) A lateral view radiograph of the colon after a barium enema in a 3-year old girl with aganglionic megacolon (Hirschsprung's disease). The upper segment of normal colon (*) is distended with fecal material. The distal segment of the colon (**) is narrow and is the portion of colon where the myenteric plexus of ganglion cells is absent. (A, Courtesy of Dr. S. Shaw, Department of Surgery, University of Virginia. From Sadler TW: *Langman's Medical Embryology*, 7th ed. Baltimore, Williams & Wilkins, 1995, p 264; B, From Wyllie R: Congenital aganglionic megacolon [Hirschsprung's disease]. In Behrman RE, Kliegman RM, Jenson HB [eds]: *Nelson Textbook of Pediatrics*, 16th ed. Philadelphia, WB Saunders, 1999.)

IV. HINGUT DERIVATIVES are supplied by the **inferior mesenteric artery.**

    A. Distal third of the transverse colon, descending colon, and sigmoid colon

        1. Formation. The cranial end of the hindgut forms the distal third of the transverse colon, descending colon, and sigmoid colon.

        2. Clinical correlations. Aganglionic megacolon (Hirschsprung's disease) results from the failure of neural crest cells to form the myenteric plexus in the sigmoid colon and rectum. (See **Figure 7-2B.**) This condition is associated with the loss of peristalsis, fecal retention, and abdominal distention.

    B. Rectum and upper anal canal. The terminal end of the hindgut is a pouch called the **cloaca.** The cloaca is partitioned by the **urorectal septum** into the rectum, upper anal canal, and urogenital sinus **(Figure 7-3A, B).**

V. ANAL CANAL

    A. Formation. The upper anal canal is a hindgut derivative, whereas the **lower anal canal**

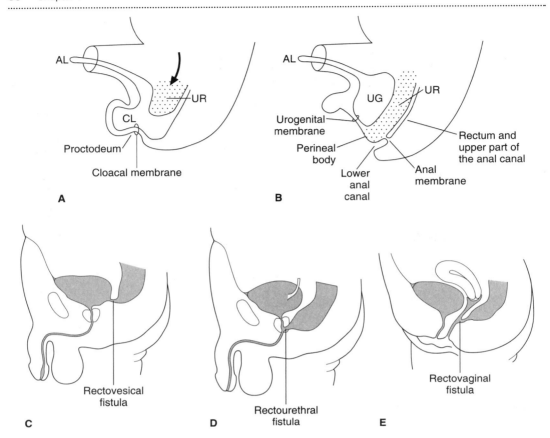

Figure 7-3. (*A, B*) Partitioning of the cloaca. The cloaca (CL) is partitioned into the rectum and upper anal canal and urogenital sinus (UG) by the urorectal septum (UR). The *arrow* indicates the direction of growth of the UR toward the body surface where it fuses at the perineal body. The surface ectoderm invaginates to form the proctodeum, which eventually forms the lower anal canal. The upper and lower anal canal meet at the anal membrane. *AL* = allantois. (*C, D, E*) Defects associated with abnormal UR septum formation. (*C*) Rectovesical fistula. (*D*) A rectourethral fistula, which generally occurs in males, is associated with the prostatic urethra and is sometimes called a rectoprostatic fistula. (*E*) Rectovaginal fistula. (C–E redrawn from Larsen WJ: *Human Embryology*, 2nd ed. New York, Churchill Livingstone, 1997, p 268.)

develops from an envagination of surface **ectoderm** called the **proctodeum.** The junction between the upper and lower anal canal forms the **anal membrane** and is marked in the adult by the **pectinate line.**

B. Clinical correlations (see Figure 7-3 C, D, E)

    1. **Anorectal agenesis** occurs when the rectum ends as a blind sac **above** the puborectalis muscle owing to abnormal formation of the urorectal septum. This condition may be accompanied by a **rectovesical fistula, rectourethral fistula,** or **rectovaginal fistula.**

    2. **Anal agenesis** occurs when the anal canal ends as a blind sac **below** the puborec-

Table 7-1

Derivation of Adult Mesenteries

Embryonic Mesentery	Adult Mesentery
Ventral mesentery	Lesser omentum (hepatoduodenal and hepatogastric ligaments), falciform ligament, coronary ligament, and triangular ligament
Dorsal mesentery	Greater omentum (gastrorenal, gastrosplenic, gastrocolic, and splenorenal ligaments), mesentery of the small intestine, mesoappendix, transverse mesocolon, sigmoid mesocolon

talis muscle owing to abnormal formation of the urorectal septum. This condition may also be accompanied by a **rectovesical fistula, rectourethral fistula,** or **rectovaginal fistula.**

VI. MESENTERIES. The primitive gut tube is suspended within the peritoneal cavity of the embryo by a **ventral** and **dorsal mesentery** from which all adult mesenteries are derived (**Table 7-1**).

8

Urinary System

I. OVERVIEW (Figure 8-1). **Intermediate mesoderm** forms a longitudinal elevation along the dorsal body wall called the **nephrogenic cord,** which forms the **pronephros, mesonephros, and metanephros (adult kidney).** The homeobox genes, **Lim-1** and **Pax-2,** appear to be important in this early stage of kidney development.

    A. The **pronephros** is not functional and completely regresses.

    B. The **mesonephros** is functional for a short period and completely regresses, except for the **mesonephric (wolffian) duct.**

    C. The **metanephros (adult kidney)** develops from two different sources:

        1. The **ureteric bud** is an outgrowth of the mesonephric duct. This outgrowth is regulated by **WT-1** (an anti-oncogene), **GDNF** (glial cell line–derived neurotrophic factor), and **c-Ret** (a tyrosine kinase receptor).

        2. The **metanephric mesoderm** is a condensation of mesoderm near the ureteric bud.

II. DEVELOPMENT OF THE KIDNEY (Table 8-1 and Figure 8-2)

    A. Development of the metanephros

        1. The ureteric bud penetrates the metanephric mesoderm and undergoes repeated divisions to form the **collecting duct, minor calyx, major calyx, renal pelvis, and ureter.**

        2. The metanephric mesoderm forms **metanephric vesicles (or blastema)** that differentiate into **primitive renal tubules.** This differentiation is regulated by **FGF-2** (fibroblast growth factor), **BMP-7** (bone morphogenetic protein), and **Wnt-11.**

        3. The primitive renal tubules eventually form the **renal glomerulus, renal (Bowman's) capsule, proximal convoluted tubule, loop of Henle, distal convoluted tubule, and connecting tubule.**

    B. Relative ascent of the kidneys

        1. The fetal metanephros is located in the sacral region, whereas the adult kidney is located at vertebral levels T12-L3. The change in location results from a disproportionate growth of the embryo caudal to the metanephros.

        2. During the relative ascent, the kidneys rotate 90 degrees medially, causing the hilum to orientate medially.

    C. Blood supply of the kidneys

        1. The blood supply changes as the metanephros undergoes its relative ascent. The

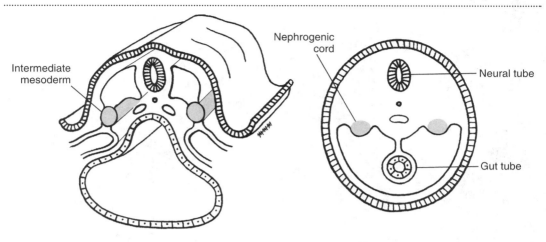

Figure 8-1.   Formation of the nephrogenic cord as the embryo goes through craniocaudal and lateral folding.

metanephros will receive its blood supply from arteries at progressively higher levels until the definitive renal arteries develop at L2.

  2. Arteries formed during the ascent may persist and are called **supernumerary arteries.** Supernumerary arteries are end arteries; therefore, damage to them will result in necrosis of kidney parenchyma.

III. DEVELOPMENT OF THE UROGENITAL SINUS (Figure 8-2A)

  A. Urinary bladder

  1. The urinary bladder develops from the upper end of the **urogenital sinus,** which is continuous with the **allantois.**

  2. The allantois normally degenerates and forms a fibrous cord in the adult called the **urachus** or **median umbilical ligament.**

Table 8-1
Development of the Kidney

Embryo	Adult Derivative
Ureteric bud	Collecting duct Minor calyx Major calyx Renal pelvis Ureter
Metanephric mesoderm	Renal glomerulus Renal (Bowman's) capsule Proximal convoluted tubule Loop of Henle Distal convoluted tubule Connecting tubule

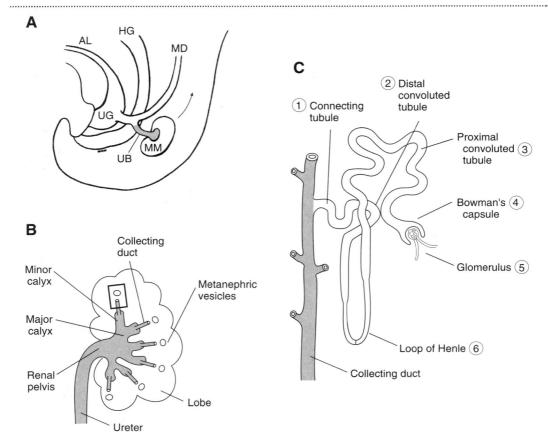

Figure 8-2. Formation of the adult kidney. (A) Lateral view of the embryo showing the ureteric bud (UB; shaded) budding off the mesonephric duct (MD) and the metanephric mesoderm (MM). The *arrow* indicates the ascent of the kidney. *AL* = allantois; *HG* = hindgut; *UG* = urogenital sinus. (B) Lateral view of a fetal kidney. *Shaded area* indicates structures formed from the ureteric bud. Note the lobulated appearance of a fetal kidney. The lobulation disappears during infancy as the kidney grows through elongation of the proximal convoluted tubules and loops of Henle. (C) Enlarged view of the rectangle shown in B, illustrating a collecting duct (*Shaded*) derived from the ureteric bud and those structures derived from the metanephric vesicle. Structures numbered ① through ⑥ make up a nephron. (B and C from Dudek RW, Fix JF: *BRS Embryology*, 2nd ed. Baltimore, Williams & Wilkins, 1998, p 165.)

     3. The **trigone of the bladder** is formed by the incorporation of the lower end of the mesonephric ducts into the posterior wall of the urogenital sinus.

  B. Inferior two thirds of the vagina (see Chapter 9, Figures 9-1 and 9-2)

     1. The paramesonephric ducts project into the dorsal wall of the urogenital sinus and induce the formation of the **sinovaginal bulbs.**

     2. The sinovaginal bulbs fuse to form the **vaginal plate,** which canalizes and develops into the inferior two thirds of the vagina.

  C. Female urethra and vestibule of the vagina

1. These are formed from the lower end of the urogenital sinus.

2. Outgrowths from these structures form the urethral, paraurethral, and greater vestibular glands.

D. Male urethra

1. The prostatic urethra, membranous urethra, and proximal part of the penile urethra form from the lower end of the urogenital sinus.

2. The distal part of the penile urethra forms from an ectodermal ingrowth called the **glandular plate,** which becomes canalized to form the **navicular fossa.**

IV. DEVELOPMENT OF THE SUPRARENAL GLAND

A. Cortex

1. The cortex forms from two episodes of mesoderm proliferation; the first episode forms the **fetal cortex,** and the second episode forms the **adult cortex.**

2. The fetal cortex is present at birth but regresses by the second postnatal month.

3. The **zona glomerulosa** and **zona fasciculata** of the adult cortex are present at birth, but the **zona reticularis** is not formed until 3 years of age.

B. Medulla

1. The medulla forms when neural crest cells aggregate at the medial aspect of the fetal cortex and eventually become surrounded by the fetal cortex.

2. The neural crest cells differentiate into **chromaffin cells.** Chromaffin cells can be found in extra suprarenal sites at birth, but these sites normally will regress completely by puberty. In a normal adult, chromaffin cells are found only in the suprarenal medulla.

V. CLINICAL CORRELATIONS

A. **Renal agenesis** occurs when the ureteric bud fails to develop.

1. Unilateral renal agenesis
   a. Unilateral renal agenesis is relatively common; therefore, a physician should never assume that a patient has two kidneys.
   b. It is more common in males.
   c. It is asymptomatic and compatible with life because the remaining kidney hypertrophies.

2. Bilateral renal agenesis
   a. Bilateral renal agenesis is relatively uncommon.
   b. It causes oligohydramnios during pregnancy, which allows the uterine wall to compress the fetus, resulting in **Potter's syndrome** (deformed limbs, wrinkly skin, and abnormal facial appearance) (see Chapter 5 III C1).
   c. It is incompatible with life unless a suitable donor is available for a kidney transplant.

B. **Horseshoe kidney (Figure 8-3A)** occurs when the inferior poles of both kidneys fuse. During the ascent, the horseshoe kidney gets trapped behind the **inferior mesenteric artery.**

C. **Urachal fistula** occurs when the allantois persists, thus forming a direct connection between the urinary bladder lumen and outside of the body at the umbilicus. This condition is associated with urine drainage from the umbilicus.

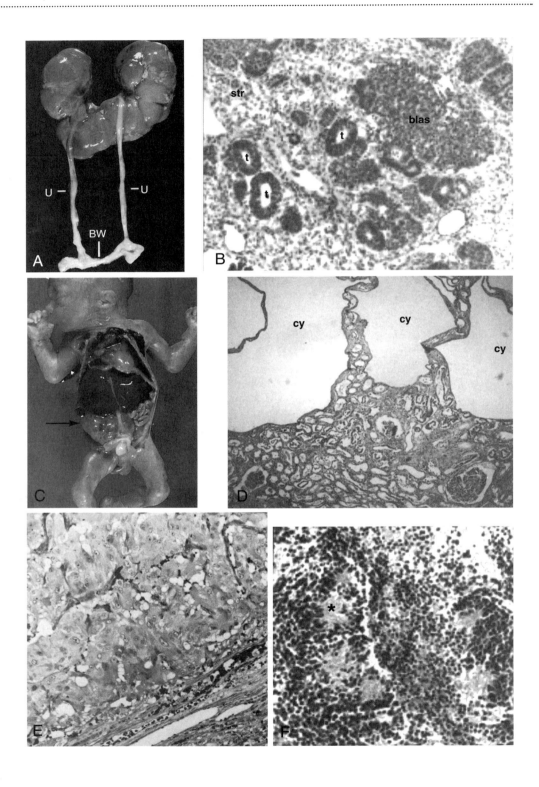

D. **Ectopic ureteric orifices**

1. **In males,** the ectopic ureter usually opens into the neck of the bladder or prostatic urethra.

2. **In females,** the ectopic ureter usually opens into the neck of the bladder or vestibule of the vagina.

3. **Incontinence** is the common complaint because urine continually dribbles from the urethra in males and from the urethra or the vagina in females.

E. **Wilms' tumor (Figure 8-3B)**

1. Wilms' tumor is the **most common primary renal tumor of childhood.**

2. The tumor presents as a large, solitary, well-circumscribed mass that on cut section is soft, homogeneous, and tan to gray.

3. Wilms' tumor is interesting histologically, because this tumor tends to recapitulate different stages of embryologic formation of the kidney. **Three classic histologic areas** are described: (1) a stromal area, (2) a blastemal area of tightly packed embryonic cells, and (3) a tubular area.

F. **Polycystic disease of the kidneys (Figure 8-3 C, D)**

1. Polycystic disease of the kidneys occurs when the loops of Henle dilate, forming **large cysts** that severely compromise kidney function.

2. It is a **relatively common hereditary disease.**

3. It is associated clinically with cysts of the liver, pancreas, and lungs.

4. **Treatment** consists in dialysis and kidney transplantation.

G. **Congenital adrenal hyperplasia (CAH;** see Chapter 9 IV C1 and Figure 9-4 A)

1. CAH is caused most commonly by mutations in genes for enzymes involved in adrenocortical steroid biosynthesis (e.g., **21-hydroxylase deficiency, 11β-hydroxylase deficiency**).

2. In 21-hydroxylase deficiency (90% of all cases), there is virtually no synthesis of the aldosterone or cortisol, so that intermediates are funneled into androgen biosynthesis, thus elevating androgen levels.

3. The **elevated levels of androgens** lead to virilization of a female fetus ranging from

Figure 8-3. (A) Photograph of a horseshoe kidney. U = ureter; BW = bladder wall. (B) Photomicrograph of Wilms' tumor. This tumor is characterized histologically by recognizable attempts to recapitulate embryonic development of the kidney. In this regard, the following three components are seen: (1) metanephric blastema elements (*blas*) consisting of clumps of small, tightly packed embryonic cells; (2) stromal elements (*str*); and (3) epithelial elements, generally in the form of abortive attempts at forming tubules (*t*) or glomeruli. (C) Photograph of an infant with polycystic kidney. (D) Photomicrograph of polycystic kidney showing large, fluid-filled cysts (CY) throughout the substance of the kidney. Between the cysts, some functioning nephrons can be observed. (E) Photomicrograph of a pheochromocytoma. The neoplastic cells have abundant cytoplasm with small centrally located nuclei. The cells are generally separated into clusters separated by a slender stroma and numerous capillaries. (F) Photomicrograph of a neuroblastoma. The neoplastic cells are small, primitive-looking cells with dark nuclei and scant cytoplasm. The cells are generally arranged as solid sheets and some cells arrange around a central fibrillar area forming Homer-Wright pseudorosettes (*). (A, from Stevenson RE: *Human Malformations and Related Anomalies.* New York, Oxford University Press, 1993. C, From Papp Z: *Atlas of Fetal Diagnosis.* New York, Elsevier, 1992, p 178. B, D, E, and F, From East Carolina University, Department of Pathology slide collection.)

mild clitoral enlargement to complete labioscrotal fusion with a phalloid organ (i.e., **female pseudointersexuality**)

4. Because cortisol cannot be synthesized, negative feedback to the adenohypophysis does not occur; thus, ACTH continues to stimulate the adrenal cortex and results in adrenal hyperplasia.

5. Because aldosterone cannot be synthesized, the patient presents with **hyponatremia** ("salt-wasting") with adjoining **dehydration** and **hyperkalemia.**

6. Treatment includes immediate infusion of intravenous saline and long-term steroid hormone replacement, both cortisol and mineralocorticoids (9α-fludrocortisone).

H. Pheochromocytoma (Figure 8-3E)

1. Pheochromocytoma is a relatively rare neoplasm that contains both **epinephrine and norepinephrine.**

2. It occurs mainly in **adults 40–60 years old.**

3. It is generally found in the region of the adrenal gland, but may be found in extra suprarenal sites.

4. Associated signs and symptoms include persistent or paroxysmal hypertension, anxiety, tremor, profuse sweating, pallor, chest pain, and abdominal pain.

5. Common laboratory findings are increased urine vanillylmandelic acid (VMA) and metanephrine levels, inability to suppress catecholamines with clonidine, and hyperglycemia.

6. Treatment is by surgery or phenoxybenzamine (an α-adrenergic antagonist).

I. Neuroblastoma (Figure 8-3F)

1. Neuroblastoma is a common extracranial neoplasm containing primitive neuroblasts of neural crest origin.

2. It **occurs mainly in children.**

3. It is found in **extra-adrenal sites** usually along the sympathetic chain ganglia (60%) or within the adrenal medulla (40%).

4. It contains small cells arranged in **Homer-Wright pseudorosettes.**

5. It involves **increased urine VMA and metanephrine** levels.

6. It **metastasizes widely.**

9
Reproductive System

I. INDIFFERENT EMBRYO. Between weeks 1 and 6, female and male embryos are phenotypically indistinguishable, even though the genotype (XX or XY) of the embryo is established at fertilization. **By week 12,** some female and male characteristics of the external genitalia can be recognized. **By week 20,** phenotypic differentiation is complete.

   A. Phenotypic differentiation is determined by the **Sry gene,** which is located on the short arm of the Y chromosome.

   1. The *Sry* gene encodes for a protein called **testes-determining factor (TDF).** TDF is a 220-amino acid nonhistone protein that contains a highly conserved DNA-binding region called a high mobility group box.

   2. As the indifferent gonad develops into the testes, Leydig cells and Sertoli cells differentiate to produce **testosterone** and **müllerian-inhibiting factor (MIF),** respectively.

   3. In the presence of **TDF, testosterone, and MIF,** the indifferent embryo will be directed to a **male phenotype.**

   4. In the absence of TDF, testosterone, and MIF, the indifferent embryo will be directed to a female **phenotype.**

   B. The components of the indifferent embryo that are remodeled to form the adult female and male reproductive systems are the **gonads, paramesonephric (müllerian) duct, mesonephric (wolffian) duct and tubules, phallus, urethral folds, and genital swellings (Figure 9-1** and **Table 9-1).**

II. DESCENT OF THE OVARY AND TESTES. The ovaries and testes develop within the abdominal cavity but later descend into the pelvis and scrotum, respectively. This descent involves the **gubernaculum** (a band of fibrous tissue) and the **processus vaginalis** (an evagination of peritoneum).

   A. Ovary

   1. The gubernaculum extends from the ovary to the junction of the uterus and uterine tubes (forming the **ovarian ligament** in the adult female) and then continues into the labia majora (forming the **round ligament of the uterus** in the adult female).

   2. The processus vaginalis is obliterated in the adult female.

   B. Testes

   1. The gubernaculum extends from the testes to the genital swellings (forming the **gubernaculum testes** in the adult male, which anchors the testes within the scrotal sac).

A. The Indifferent Embryo

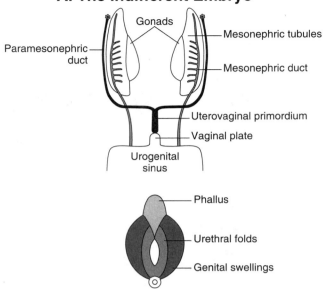

B. Female Reproductive System
C. Male Reproductive System

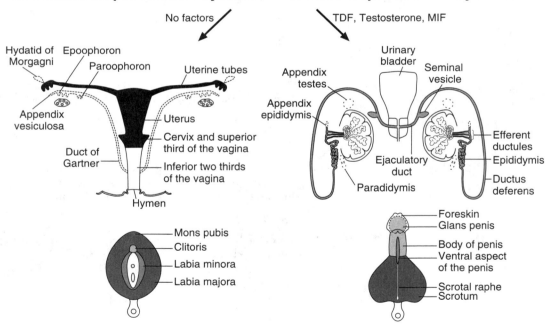

Figure 9-1. (A) The indifferent embryo, with components indicated: gonads, paramesonephric ducts, mesonephric ducts and tubules, phallus, urethral folds, genital swellings. (B) The female reproductive system. In the absence of TDF, testosterone, and MIF, the indifferent embryo will undergo phenotypic differentiation to female structures. Note that the paramesonephric duct is primarily involved in female development. The mesonephric duct and tubules form only vestigial structures in the female. (C) The male reproductive system. In the presence of TDF, testosterone, and MIF, the indifferent embryo will undergo phenotypic differentiation to male structures. Note that the mesonephric duct and tubules are primarily involved in male development. The paramesonephric ducts form only vestigial structures in the male.

Table 9-1
Development of the Adult Female and Male Reproductive Systems*

Indifferent Embryo	Adult Female	Adult Male
Gonads	Ovary, primordial follicles, rete ovarii	Testes, seminiferous tubules, tubuli recti, rete testes, Leydig cells, Sertoli cells
Paramesonephric ducts	Uterine tubes, uterus, cervix and superior third of the vagina† **Hydatid of Morgagni**	**Appendix testes**
Mesonephric ducts	**Appendix vesiculosa** **Duct of Gartner**	Epididymis, ductus deferens, seminal vesicles, ejaculatory duct **Appendix epididymis**
Mesonephric tubules	**Epoophoron, paroophoron**	Efferent ductules **Paradidymis**
Phallus	Clitoris	Glans and body of the penis
Urethral folds	Labia minora	Ventral aspect of the penis
Genital swellings	Labia majora, mons pubis	Scrotum

*__Demi italics__ indicate vestigial structures.
†The inferior two-thirds of the vagina develops from the vaginal plate of the urogenital sinus (see Chapter 8 III B).

> **2.** The processus vaginalis forms the **tunica vaginalis** in the adult male.

III. DEVELOPMENT OF THE PROSTATE GLAND

> **A.** The prostate gland develops from multiple outgrowths of the prostatic urethra.

> **B.** **Dihydrotestosterone** (DHT) is the main mediator of prostatic growth in males. This is clinically important in benign prostatic hypertrophy because **finasteride** (a 5α-reductase inhibitor) can reduce DHT levels and shrink the prostate gland. In addition, the action of DHT can be blocked by the receptor antagonist called **flutamide.**

IV. CLINICAL CORRELATIONS

> **A.** Female (Figure 9-2)

>> **1.** **Double uterus with double vagina** is a condition where two uteri and two vaginas are present. It results from the complete lack of fusion of the paramesonephric ducts and the sinovaginal bulbs.

>> **2.** **Bicornuate uterus** is a condition where the uterus has two horns entering a common vagina. It results from partial fusion of the paramesonephric ducts.

>> **3.** **Bicornuate uterus with rudimentary horn** is a condition in which only one side of the uterus forms normally. It results from retarded growth of one of the paramesonephric ducts.

>> **4.** **Atresia of the vagina** is a condition in which the vaginal lumen is blocked. It results from failure of the vaginal plate to canalize and form a lumen. When only the inferior part of the vaginal plate fails to canalize, a condition known as **imperforate hymen** occurs.

>> **5.** **Absence of uterus and vagina** results from the failure of the paramesonephric ducts and the sinovaginal bulbs to develop.

A. Formation of the Uterus and Vagina

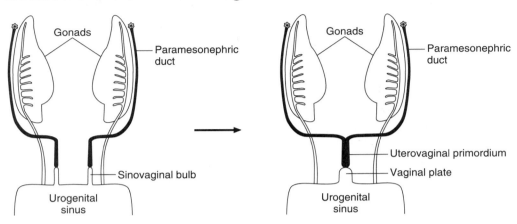

B. Congenital Anomalies

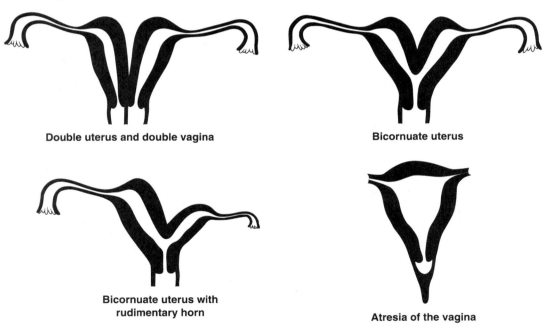

Double uterus and double vagina

Bicornuate uterus

Bicornuate uterus with rudimentary horn

Atresia of the vagina

Figure 9-2. (A) Formation of the uterus and vagina. The paramesonephric ducts fuse in the midline to form the uterovaginal primordium which develops into the uterus, cervix, and superior third of the vagina. The paramesonephric ducts project into the dorsal wall of the urogenital sinus and induce the formation of the sinovaginal bulbs. The sinovaginal bulbs fuse to form the solid vaginal plate which canalizes to form the inferior two thirds of the vagina. (B) Diagram depicting various congenital anomalies of the uterus and vagina. (From Dudek RW, Fix JF: *BRS Embryology*, 2nd ed. Baltimore, Williams & Wilkins, 1998, p 179.)

B. Male

1. Hypospadias (Figure 9-3) occurs when the urethral folds fail to fuse completely, resulting in the external urethral orifice opening onto the ventral surface of the penis. It is generally associated with a poorly developed penis that curves ventrally, known as **chordee (Figure 9-3B).**

2. Epispadias (Figure 9-3C) occurs when the external urethral orifice opens onto the dorsal surface of the penis. It is generally associated with **exstrophy of the bladder.**

3. Undescended testes (cryptorchidism; Figure 9-3D) occurs when the testes fail to descend into the scrotum. This normally is evident within 3 months after birth. The undescended testes may be found in the abdominal cavity or in the inguinal canal. Bilateral cryptorchidism results in **sterility.**

4. Hydrocele of the testes (Figure 9-3E) occurs when a small patency of the processus vaginalis remains so that peritoneal fluid can flow into the tunica vaginalis, which results in a fluid-filled cyst near the testes.

5. Congenital inguinal hernia occurs when a large patency of the processus vaginalis remains so that a loop of intestine may herniate into the scrotum or labia majora. It is most common in males and is generally associated with **cryptorchidism.**

C. Other

1. Female pseudointersexuality **(Figure 9-4A)**
   a. This occurs when an individual has only ovarian tissue histologically and masculinization of the female external genitalia. These individuals have a 46,XX genotype.
   b. The most common cause is **congenital adrenal hyperplasia,** a condition in which the fetus produces excess androgens (see Chapter 8 V G).

2. Male pseudointersexuality **(see Figure 9-4B)**
   a. This occurs when an individual has only testicular tissue histologically and various stages of stunted development of the male external genitalia. Individuals have a 46,XY genotype.
   b. The most common cause is **inadequate production of testosterone and MIF** by the fetal testes, owing to the following deficiencies:
   (1) 5α-Reductase 2 deficiency
      (a) Causes. A mutation in the **5α-reductase 2 gene** renders 5α-reductase 2 enzyme inactive. Normally, 5α-reductase 2 catalyzes the conversion of testosterone (T) to DHT.
      (b) Clinical findings. Underdevelopment of the penis and scrotum (microphallus, hypospadias, and bifid scrotum) and prostate gland is evident. The epididymis, ductus deferens, seminal vesicle, and ejaculatory duct are normal. These clinical findings have led to the inference that DHT is essential in the development of the penis and scrotum (external genitalia) and prostate gland in the genotypic XY fetus. At puberty, these individuals demonstrate a **striking virilization.**
      (c) Laboratory tests. An increased **T:DHT ratio** is diagnostic (normal = 5; 5α-reductase 2 deficiency = 20–60).
   (2) 17β-Hydroxysteroid dehydrogenase 3 (HSD) deficiency
      (a) Causes. A mutation in the **17β HSD 3 gene** renders 17β HSD 3 enzyme inactive. Normally, 17β HSD 3 catalyzes the conversion of androstenedione to testosterone.

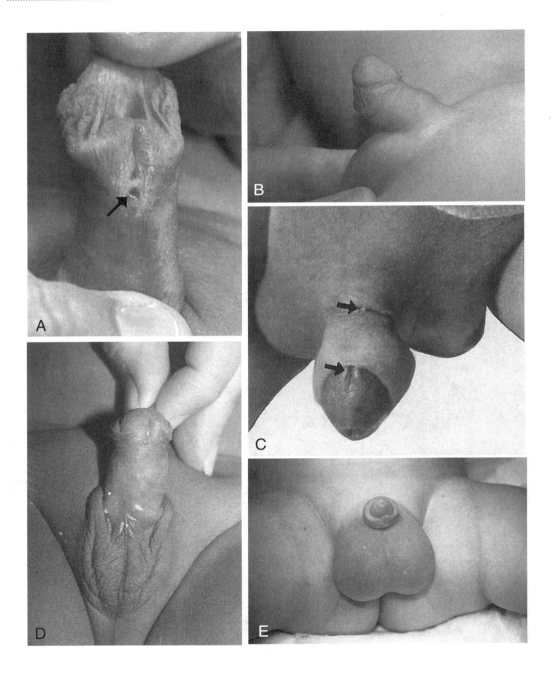

Figure 9-3. (A) Hypospadias with urethral opening on ventral surface (*arrow*). (B) Chordee. Note that the penis is poorly developed and bowed ventrally. (C) Epispadias with two urethral openings on the dorsal surface of the penis (*arrows*). (D) Cryptorchidism. Note that the both testes have not descended into the scrotal sac. (E) Bilateral hydrocele. (B and E courtesy of Dr. T. Ernesto Figueroa. All views from Gilbert-Barness ES [ed]: *Potter's Atlas of Fetal and Infant Pathology.* St. Louis, CV Mosby, 1998, p 294.)

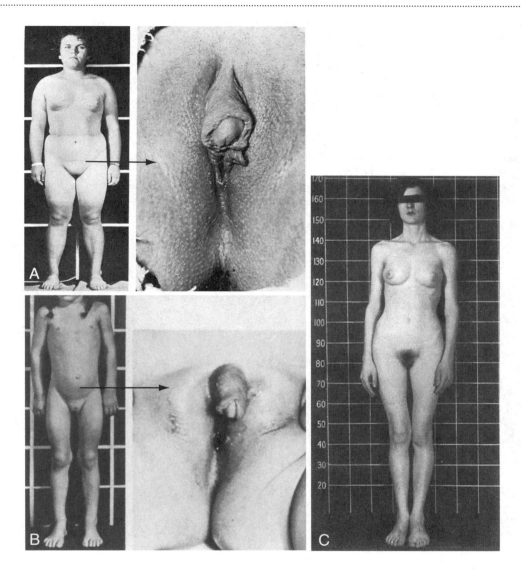

Figure 9-4.   (A) A patient (XX genotype) with female pseudointersexuality due to congenital adrenal hyperplasia (see Chapter 8 V G). Masculinization of female external genitalia is apparent with fusion of the labia majora and enlarged clitoris. (B) A patient (XY genotype) with male pseudointersexuality. Stunted development of male external genitalia is apparent. The stunted external genitalia fooled the parents and the physician into thinking that this XY infant was a girl. In fact, this child was raised as a girl (note the pigtails). As this child neared puberty, testosterone levels increased and clitoral enlargement ensued. This alarmed the parents and the child was brought in for clinical evaluation. (C) A patient (XY genotype) with complete androgen insensitivity (CAIS or testicular feminization). Complete feminization of the male external genitalia is apparent. (A, Courtesy of Dr. J. Kitchin, Department of Obstetrics and Gynecology, University of Virginia; from Sadler TW: *Langman's Medical Embryology,* 7th ed. Baltimore, Williams & Wilkins, 1995, p 305. B, From Warkany J: *Congenital Malformations: Notes and Comments.* Chicago, Year Book Medical Publishers, 1971, p 337. C, From Jones HW, Scott WW: *Hermaphroditism, Genital Anomalies and Related Endocrine Disorders.* Baltimore, Williams & Wilkins, 1958.)

    (b) **Clinical findings.** Underdevelopment of the penis and scrotum (microphallus, hypospadias, and bifid scrotum) and prostate gland is evident. The epididymis, ductus deferens, seminal vesicle, and ejaculatory duct are normal. The clinical findings in 17β-HSD deficiency and 5α-reductase 2 deficiency are very similar.

3. **Complete androgen insensitivity (CAIS; testicular feminization syndrome; Figure 9-4C)**

    a. CAIS occurs when a fetus with a 46,XY genotype develops testes and female external genitalia with a rudimentary vagina; uterus and uterine tubes are generally absent. Testes may be found in the labia majora (they are surgically removed to circumvent malignant tumor formation).

    b. Individuals with this syndrome present as **normal-appearing females,** and their psychosocial orientation is female despite their genotype.

    c. The most common cause is a mutation in the **androgen receptor (AR) gene** that renders AR inactive.

10

Respiratory System

I. OVERVIEW (Figure 10-1)

A. The first sign of respiratory system development is the formation of a **respiratory diverticulum** in the ventral wall of the foregut.

B. The distal end of the respiratory diverticulum enlarges to form the **lung bud.**

C. The lung bud divides into two **bronchial buds** that branch into the **primary, secondary,** and **tertiary bronchi.**

D. The respiratory diverticulum is initially in open communication with the foregut, but eventually this communication is obliterated by the formation of the **tracheoesophageal septum,** which separates the trachea from the esophagus.

E. The **Hox complex, FGF-10** (fibroblast growth factor), **BMP-4** (bone morphogenetic protein), **N-*myc*** (a proto-oncogene), **syndecan** (a proteoglycan), **tenasin** (an extracellular matrix protein), and **epimorphin** (a protein) appear to play a role in the development of the respiratory system.

II. DEVELOPMENT OF THE TRACHEA

A. **Formation.** The respiratory diverticulum elongates considerably before the bronchial buds appear. This elongated portion of the respiratory diverticulum forms the trachea.

B. **Clinical correlation: tracheoesophageal fistula (Figure 10-2)**

   1. **Definition.** Tracheoesophageal fistula is an abnormal communication (fistula) between the trachea and the esophagus, which is caused by improper formation of the tracheoesophageal septum. It is generally associated with **esophageal atresia and polyhydramnios.** The most common type (90% of all cases) is esophageal atresia with a fistula between the esophagus and the **distal one-third of the trachea.**

   2. **Clinical features** include excessive accumulation of saliva or mucus in the infant's nose and mouth; episodes of gagging and cyanosis after swallowing milk; abdominal distention after crying; and reflux of gastric contents into the lungs, causing pneumonitis.

   3. **Diagnostic features** include the inability to pass a catheter into the stomach and radiographs demonstrating air in the infant's stomach.

III. DEVELOPMENT OF THE BRONCHI

A. Formation

   1. The lung bud divides into two bronchial buds.

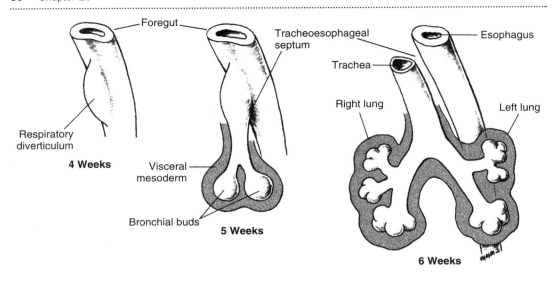

Figure 10-1.   Development of the respiratory system at weeks 4–6.

2. In week 5 of development, bronchial buds enlarge to form **primary bronchi.** The right primary bronchus is larger and more vertical than the left primary bronchus; this relationship persists throughout adult life and accounts for the greater likelihood of foreign bodies lodging on the right side than on the left.

3. Primary bronchi further subdivide into **secondary bronchi** (three on the right side and two on the left side, corresponding to the lobes of the adult lung).

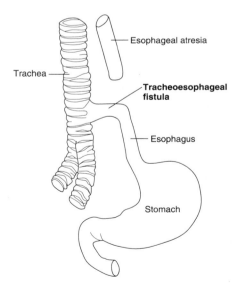

Figure 10-2.   Tracheoesophageal fistula. In 90% of these cases, there is esophageal atresia with a fistula between the esophagus and the distal one-third of the trachea.

4. Secondary bronchi further subdivide into **tertiary (or segmental) bronchi** (10 on the right side and 8 or 9 on the left side). These are the primordia of the **bronchopulmonary segments.**

5. As the bronchi develop, they expand laterally and caudally into a space known as the primitive pleural cavity; visceral mesoderm covering the outside of the bronchi develops into **visceral pleura,** and somatic mesoderm covering the inside of the body wall develops into **parietal pleura.**

B. Clinical correlations

1. Bronchopulmonary segment. This segment of lung tissue is supplied by a tertiary (segmental) bronchus. Surgeons can resect diseased lung tissue along bronchopulmonary segments rather than removing the entire lobe.

2. Congenital neonatal emphysema is an overdistention with air of one or more lobes of the lung. Emphysema is caused by collapsed bronchi due to failure of bronchial cartilage to develop. Air can be inspired through collapsed bronchi, but cannot be expired.

3. Congenital bronchial cysts (bronchiectasis) are caused by dilatation of the bronchi. Cysts may be solitary or multiple and can be filled with air or fluid. Multiple cysts demonstrate a honeycomb appearance on a radiograph. The honeycomb appearance may be a useful diagnostic tool on a radiograph.

IV. DEVELOPMENT OF THE LUNGS (Figure 10-3 and Table 10-1)

A. Formation. The lungs undergo four periods of development: the **glandular period, canalicular period, terminal sac period,** and **alveolar period.**

B. Clinical correlations

1. Aeration at birth
   a. Aeration is the replacement of fluid by air in the newborn's lungs. At birth, the lungs are half-filled with fluid derived from the lungs (main source), amniotic cavity, and tracheal glands. The fluid is eliminated at birth through the nose and mouth during delivery, and later through resorption by pulmonary capillaries and lymphatics.
   b. The lungs of a stillborn baby will sink when placed in water, because they contain fluid rather than air.

2. Pulmonary agenesis involves the complete absence of lungs, bronchi, and vasculature. This rare condition is caused by failure of bronchial buds to develop. **Unilateral pulmonary agenesis** is compatible with life.

3. Pulmonary hypoplasia involves a poorly developed bronchial tree with abnormal histology. It may be partial (involving a small segment of lung) or total (involving the entire lung). It can be found in association with:
   a. A **congenital diaphragmatic hernia** (i.e., a herniation of abdominal contents into the thorax compresses the developing lung; see Chapter 15).
   b. **Bilateral renal agenesis** (see Chapter 8 V A), which causes an insufficient amount of amniotic fluid (**oligohydramnios;** see Chapter 5 III C) to be produced, which in turn increases pressure on the fetal thorax.

4. Respiratory distress syndrome (RDS) is caused by a deficiency or absence of **surfactant.** This surface-active detergent consists of **phosphatidylcholine** (mainly **dipalmitoyl lecithin**) and **proteins;** it coats the inside of alveoli and maintains alveolar patency.

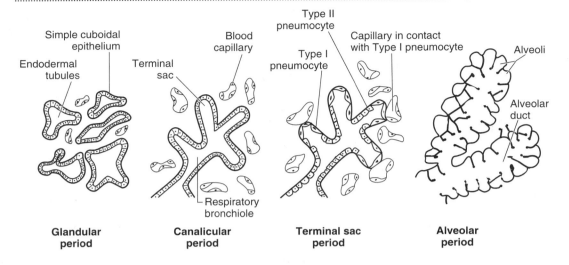

| Glandular period | Canalicular period | Terminal sac period | Alveolar period |

Figure 10-3.   Histologic appearance of lung tissue during the four time periods of lung development.

During the glandular period, the developing lung resembles the branching of a compound exocrine gland into a bush-like array of endodermal tubules, which comprise the air-conducting system. However, histologic structures involved in gas exchange are not yet formed, and respiration is not possible.

During the canalicular period, respiratory bronchioles and terminal sacs (primitive alveoli) develop. Vascularization increases owing to the formation of capillaries in visceral mesoderm that surround the respiratory bronchioles and terminal sacs.

During the terminal sac period, the number of terminal sacs and vascularization increases greatly. Differentiation of type I pneumocytes (thin, flat cells that make up part of the blood–air barrier) and type II pneumocytes (which produce surfactant) begins. Capillaries make contact with type I pneumocytes, which permits respiration and establishes the blood-air barrier.

The alveolar period begins at birth. The increase in size of the lung after birth is caused by the increased number of respiratory bronchioles and terminal sacs. Subsequently, terminal sacs develop into mature alveolar ducts and alveoli. By age 8, the adult complement of 300 million alveoli is reached.

(From Dudek RW, Fix JD: *BRS Embryology,* 2nd ed. Baltimore, Williams & Wilkins, 1998, p 142.)

Table 10-1

Stages of Lung Development

Stage	Time Period	Characteristics
Glandular	Weeks 5–17	Respiration is not possible. Premature fetuses cannot survive.
Canalicular	Weeks 16–25	Respiratory bronchioles and terminal sacs form. Vascularization increases. Premature fetuses born before week 20 rarely survive.
Terminal sac	Week 24–birth	Types I and II pneumocytes are present. Respiration is possible. Premature fetuses born between weeks 25 and 28 can survive with intensive care.
Alveolar	Birth–year 8	Respiratory bronchioles, terminal sacs, alveolar ducts, and alveoli increase in number. On chest radiograph, the lungs of a newborn infant are denser than are those of an adult because there are fewer alveoli.

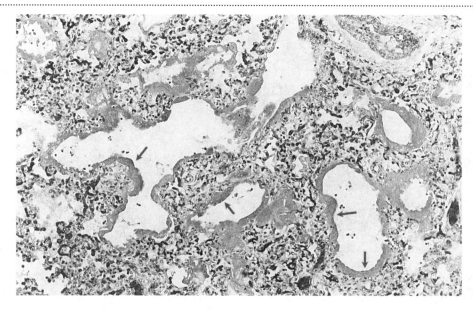

Figure 10-4.   Photomicrograph of hyaline membrane disease. The air-filled bronchioles and alveolar ducts are widely dilated. In addition, they are lined by a homogeneous hyaline material (*arrows*) that consists of fibrin and necrotic cells. Note the presence of atelectasis (i.e., the collapse of distal alveoli).

 a. **Thyroxine** and **cortisol** increase the production of surfactant.

 b. Prolonged intrauterine asphyxia decreases the production of surfactant by permanently damaging type II pneumocytes.

 c. RDS is common in premature infants and in the infants of diabetic mothers.

 d. RDS accounts for 50%–70% of deaths in premature infants.

 e. Not only does RDS threaten the infant with immediate asphyxiation, but it can also bring about **hyaline membrane disease (Figure 10-4).** Repeated gasping inhalations can damage the alveolar lining and cause hyaline membrane disease. Hyaline membrane disease is characterized histologically by collapsed alveoli (atelectasis) that contain an eosinophilic fluid that resembles a hyaline or glassy membrane.

11

Head and Neck

I. PHARYNGEAL APPARATUS (Figure 11-1) consists of pharyngeal **arches, pouches, grooves,** and **membranes,** all of which contribute greatly to the formation of the head and neck region. The **Hox complex** and **retinoic acid** appear to be important in the early stages of head and neck development. A lack or excess of retinoic acid causes striking facial anomalies.

   A. **Pharyngeal arches (1, 2, 3, 4, 6)*** contain **mesoderm** (somitomeric) and **neural crest cells.** In general, the mesoderm differentiates into **muscles** and **arteries** (i.e., aortic arches 1–6; see Chapter 6 III A), whereas neural crest cells differentiate into **bones.** In addition, each arch has a cranial nerve associated with it. **Table 11-1** summarizes the adult derivatives of the pharyngeal arches.

   B. **Pharyngeal pouches (1, 2, 3, 4)** are evaginations of endoderm that lines the foregut (Table 11-2).

   C. **Pharyngeal grooves (1, 2, 3, 4)** are invaginations of surface ectoderm. Pharyngeal groove 1 gives rise to the **epithelial lining of the external auditory meatus,** whereas all other grooves are obliterated (see Table 11-2).

   D. **Pharyngeal membranes (1, 2, 3, 4)** are located at the junction of each pharyngeal groove and pouch. Pharyngeal membrane 1 gives rise to the **tympanic membrane,** whereas all other membranes are obliterated (see Table 11-2).

II. THYROID GLAND (Figure 11-1). This gland develops from the **thyroid diverticulum,** which forms in the floor of the foregut. The thyroid diverticulum migrates caudally down the **midline** to its adult anatomic position but remains connected to the foregut via the **thyroglossal duct,** which is later obliterated. The former site of the thyroglossal duct is in-dicated in the adult by the **foramen cecum.**

III. TONGUE (Figure 11-2)

   A. **Anterior two thirds (oral part) of the tongue**

   1. The oral part of the tongue forms from the **median tongue bud and two distal tongue buds** associated with pharyngeal arch 1. The distal tongue buds overgrow the median tongue bud and fuse in the midline, forming the **median sulcus.**

   2. The oral part of the tongue is characterized by filiform papillae (no taste buds), fungiform papillae (taste buds present), and circumvallate papillae (taste buds present).

---

*Pharyngeal arch 5 degenerates in humans.

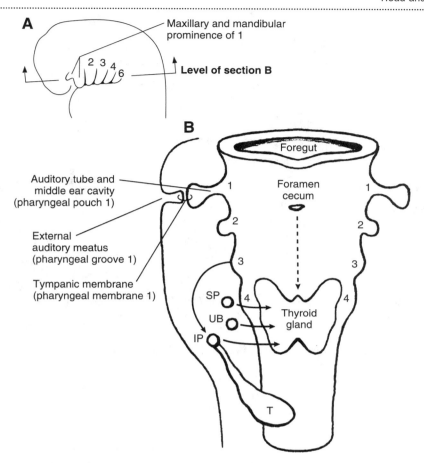

Figure 11-1.   (A) Lateral view of an embryo in week 4 of development, showing the pharyngeal arches. Note that pharyngeal arch 1 consists of a maxillary and mandibular prominence, which may cause some confusion in numbering of the arches. (B) Migration of the superior (SP) and inferior (IP) parathyroid glands, thymus (T), ultimobranchial body (UB), and thyroid gland (T). Note that the parathyroid tissue derived from pouch 3 is carried further caudally by the descent of the thymus than parathyroid tissue from pouch 4. The foramen cecum evaginates to form the thyroid diverticulum, which migrates caudally along the midline (*dotted arrow*). In addition, pharyngeal pouch 1, pharyngeal membrane 1, and pharyngeal groove 1 are shown to give rise to structures of the adult ear. *2* = pharyngeal pouch 2; *3* = pharyngeal pouch 3; *4* = pharyngeal pouch 4.

    3. **General sensation** from the mucosa is carried by the **lingual branch of the trigeminal nerve** (CN V).

    4. **Taste sensation** from the mucosa is carried by the **chorda tympani branch of the facial nerve** (CN VII).

  B. Posterior third (pharyngeal part) of the tongue

    1. The posterior third of the tongue forms from the **copula and hypobranchial eminence,** which is associated with pharyngeal arches 2, 3, and 4. The hypobranchial eminence overgrows the copula, thus eliminating any contribution of pharyngeal arch 2 in the formation of the definitive adult tongue. The line of fusion between the oral and pharyngeal parts of the tongue is indicated by the **terminal sulcus.**

Table 11-1
Adult Derivatives of the Pharyngeal Arches

Arch	Nerve	Adult Derivatives
1	CN V	*Mesoderm:* Muscles of mastication, mylohyoid, anterior belly of digastric, tensor veli palatini, tensor tympani
		Neural crest cells: Maxilla, zygomatic bone, squamous portion of the temporal bone, palatine bone, vomer, mandible, incus, malleus, sphenomandibular ligament
2	CN VII	*Mesoderm:* Muscles of facial expression, posterior belly of the digastric, stylohyoid, stapedius
		Neural crest cells: Stapes, styloid process, stylohyoid ligament, lesser horn and upper body of hyoid bone
3	CN IX	*Mesoderm:* Stylopharyngeus, common carotid arteries, internal carotid arteries
		Neural crest cells: Greater horn and lower body of the hyoid bone
4	CN X (superior laryngeal branch)	*Mesoderm:* Muscles of the soft palate (except tensor veli palatini), muscles of the pharynx (except stylopharyngeus), cricothyroid, cricopharyngeus, laryngeal cartilages, right subclavian artery, arch of the aorta
		Neural crest cells: None
6	CN X recurrent laryngeal branch)	*Mesoderm:* Intrinsic muscles of larynx (except the cricothyroid), upper muscles of the esophagus, laryngeal cartilages, pulmonary arteries, ductus arteriosus
		Neural crest cells: None

2. The posterior third of the tongue is characterized by the lingual tonsil; the lingual tonsil, palatine tonsil, and pharyngeal tonsil (adenoids) are collectively called **Waldeyer's ring,** which protects the oral port of entry.

Table 11-2
Adult Derivatives of the Pharyngeal Pouches, Grooves, and Membranes

Pouch	Adult Derivatives
1	Epithelial lining of the auditory tube and middle ear cavity
2	Epithelial lining of the palatine tonsil crypts
3	Inferior parathyroid gland and thymus
4	Superior parathyroid gland and ultimobranchial body*
Groove	
1	Epithelial lining of the external auditory meatus
2, 3, 4	Obliterated
Membrane	
1	Tympanic membrane
2, 3, 4	Obliterated

*Neural crest cells migrate into the ultimobranchial body to form parafollicular cells (C cells) of the thyroid, which secrete calcitonin.

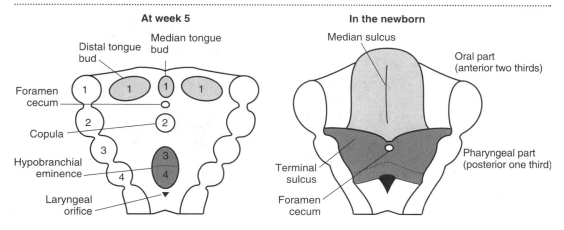

Figure 11-2. Development of the tongue. (A) At week 5. (B) In the newborn. (Adapted from Dudek RW, Fix JD: *BRS Embryology,* 2nd ed. Baltimore, Williams & Wilkins, 1998, p 153.)

    3. General sensation from the mucosa is carried primarily by the **glossopharyngeal nerve** (CN IX).

    4. Taste sensation from the mucosa is carried predominantly by the **glossopharyngeal nerve** (CN IX).

C. Muscles of the tongue

    1. The **intrinsic muscles** and **extrinsic muscles** (styloglossus, hyoglossus, genioglossus, and palatoglossus) are derived from myoblasts that migrate into the tongue region from **occipital somites.**

    2. Motor innervation for all muscles of the tongue is supplied by the **hypoglossal nerve** (CN XII), except for the palatoglossus muscle, which is innervated by the vague nerve (CN X).

IV. FACE (Figure 11-3)

A. The face is formed by three swellings: the **frontonasal prominence, maxillary prominence** (pharyngeal arch 1), and **mandibular prominence** (pharyngeal arch 1).

B. Bilateral ectodermal thickenings called **nasal placodes** develop on the ventrolateral aspects of the frontonasal prominence.

C. The nasal placodes invaginate into the underlying mesoderm to form the **nasal pits,** thus producing a ridge of tissue that forms the **medial** and **lateral nasal prominences.**

D. The **nasolacrimal groove** forms between the maxillary prominence and the lateral nasal prominence and eventually forms the **nasolacrimal duct** and **lacrimal sac.**

V. PALATE (Figure 11-4)

A. Intermaxillary segment

    1. The intermaxillary segment forms when the medial growth of the maxillary prominences causes the two medial nasal prominences to fuse together at the midline.

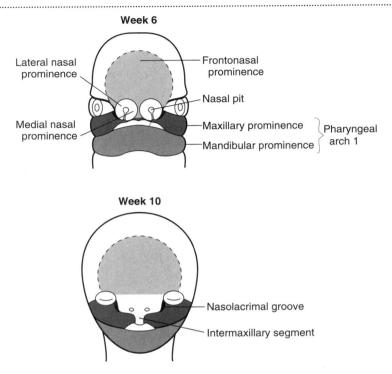

Figure 11-3. Development of the face. Note that pharyngeal arch 1 plays a major role. (Adapted from Dudek RW, Fix JD: *BRS Embryology*, 2nd ed. Baltimore, Williams & Wilkins, 1998, p 154.)

   2. The **philtrum of the lip, four incisor teeth,** and **primary palate** in the adult are formed from this segment.

B. Secondary palate

   1. The secondary palate forms from outgrowths of the maxillary prominences called the **palatine shelves.**

   2. Initially, the palatine shelves project downward on either side of the tongue but later attain a horizontal position and fuse along the midline **palatine raphe** to form the **secondary palate.**

   3. The primary and secondary palate fuse at the **incisive foramen** to form the definitive adult **palate.**

   4. Bone develops in both the primary palate and the anterior part of the secondary palate.

   5. Bone does not develop in the posterior part of the secondary palate, which eventually forms the **soft palate** and **uvula.**

   6. The **nasal septum** develops from the medial nasal prominences and fuses with the definitive palate.

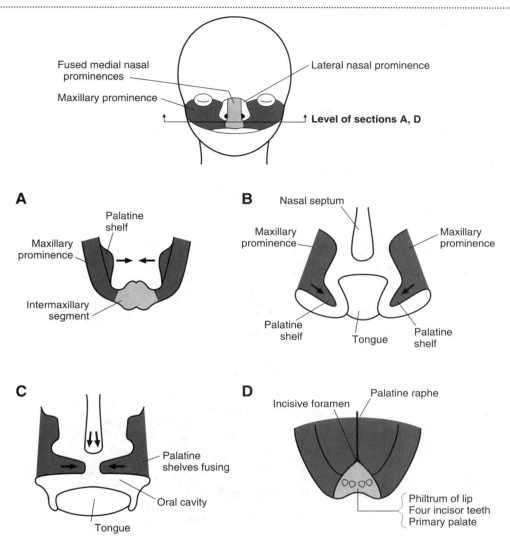

Figure 11-4. Development of the palate. (A) This horizontal section shows the intermaxillary segment and maxillary prominence with palatine shelves growing toward the midline (*arrows*). (B, C) Coronal sections showing the movements of the palatine shelves (*single arrows*) and fusion with the nasal septum (*double arrows*). (D) A horizontal section (as indicated) of the adult palate. (Level of sections in A–D is noted in top drawing.) (Adapted from Dudek RW, Fix JD: *BRS Embryology*, 2nd ed. Baltimore, Williams & Wilkins, 1998, p 155–156.)

VI. CLINICAL CORRELATIONS

A. First arch syndromes are caused by a lack of migration of neural crest cells into pharyngeal arch 1. They produce various facial anomalies. Two well-described first arch syndromes are **Treacher Collins syndrome (Figure 11-5 A)** and **Pierre Robin syndrome.**

B. DiGeorge syndrome occurs when pharyngeal pouches 3 and 4 fail to differentiate,

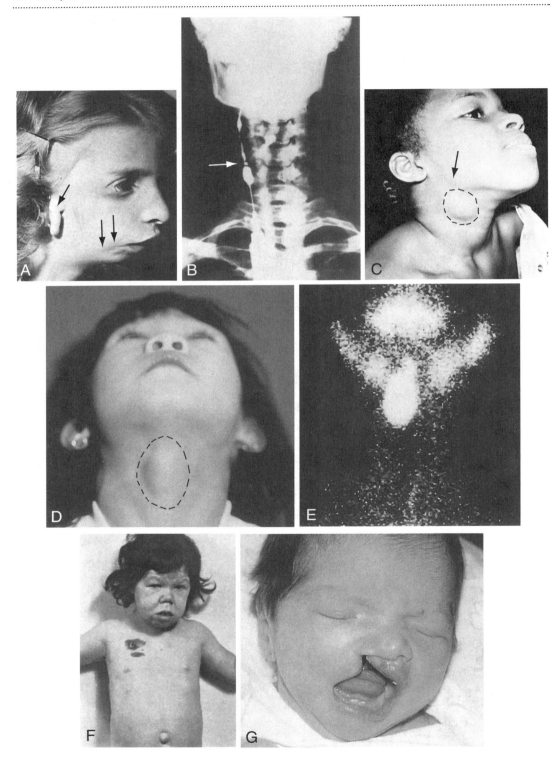

leading to the absence of the thymus and parathyroid glands. This syndrome is usually accompanied by facial anomalies that resemble first arch syndrome and cardiovascular anomalies that are caused by abnormal neural crest cell migration during the formation of the aorticopulmonary septum.

C. Pharyngeal fistula (Figure 11-5 B) occurs when pharyngeal pouch 2 and pharyngeal groove 2 persist, forming a patent opening from the internal tonsillar area to the external neck. A pharyngeal fistula is generally found along the **anterior border of the sternocleidomastoid muscle.**

D. Pharyngeal cyst (Figure 11-5 C). A pharyngeal cyst occurs when parts of the pharyngeal grooves that are normally obliterated persist, forming a cyst. This type of cyst is generally found near the **angle of the mandible.**

E. Ectopic thymus, parathyroid, and **thyroid tissue (Figure 11-5 D, E)** result from the abnormal migration of the glands from their embryonic position to their definitive adult location. Ectopic thymus and parathyroid tissue can be found in the lateral area of the neck, whereas ectopic thyroid tissue can be found along the midline.

F. Thyroglossal duct cyst. This type of cyst occurs when parts of the thyroglossal duct persist and form a cyst. A thyroglossal duct cyst is most commonly located in the midline near the hyoid bone but may also be located at the base of the tongue (it is then called a **lingual cyst).**

G. Congenital hypothyroidism (cretinism; Figure 11-5 F) occurs when a thyroid deficiency exists during the early fetal period due to either a severe lack of dietary iodine, thyroid agenesis, or mutations involving the biosynthesis of thyroid hormone.

1. This condition causes **impaired skeletal growth** and **mental retardation.**

2. This condition is characterized by dry, rough skin, wide-set eyes, periorbital puffiness, a flat broad nose, and a large protuberant tongue.

H. Ankyloglossia (tongue-tie) occurs when the frenulum of the tongue extends to the tip of the tongue, thus preventing protrusion.

I. Cleft palate (Figure 11-5 G) has many causes. It is classified as anterior or posterior. (Note that the anatomic landmark that separates anterior cleft palate defects from posterior cleft palate defects is the incisive foramen.)

Figure 11-5. (A) **Treacher Collins syndrome** is characterized by underdevelopment of the zygomatic bones, mandibular hypoplasia (*double arrows*), lower eyelid colobomas, and malformed external ears (*arrow*). (B) **Pharyngeal fistula.** A radiograph after injection of a contrast medium demonstrating the course of the fistula through the neck (*arrow*). The fistula may begin inside the throat near the tonsils, travel through the neck, and open to the outside near the anterior border of the sternocleidomastoid muscle. (C) **Pharyngeal cyst.** A fluid-filled cyst (*dotted circle*) near the angle of the mandible (*arrow*). (D, E) **Ectopic thyroid tissue.** A sublingual thyroid mass (*dotted circle*) is seen in a 5-year-old euthyroid girl. A ^{99m}Tc pertechnetate scan localizes the position and extent of the sublingual thyroid gland. There is no evidence of functioning thyroid tissue in the lower neck (i.e., normal anatomic position). (F) **Congenital hypothyroidim (cretinism).** This child shows impaired skeletal growth and mental retardation. Note the dry, rough skin (myxedema) and the protuberant tongue. (G) **Unilateral cleft lip and cleft palate.** (A, From Smith DW: *Recognizable Patterns of Human Malformation: Genetic Embryologic and Clinical Aspects,* 3rd ed. Philadelphia, WB Saunders, 1982, p 185. B and G, From Moore KL and Persaud TVN: *The Developing Human: Clinically Oriented Embryology,* 6th ed. Philadelphia, WB Saunders, 1998, pp 228, 248. C, From Sadler TW: *Langman's Medical Embryology,* 7th ed. Baltimore, Williams & Wilkins, 1995, p 325. Courtesy of Dr. A. Shaw, Department of Surgery, University of Virginia. D and E, From Leung AKC, Wong AL, and Robson WLLM: *Ectopic thyroid gland simulating a thyroglossal duct cyst.* Can J Surg 38:87, 1995. F, From Warkany J: *Congenital Malformations: Notes and Comments.* Chicago, Year Book Medical Publishers, 1971, Fig 44.4.)

1. **Anterior cleft palate** occurs when the palatine shelves fail to fuse with the primary palate.

2. **Posterior cleft palate** occurs when the palatine shelves fail to fuse with each other and with the nasal septum.

3. **Anteroposterior cleft palate** occurs when there is a combination of both defects.

J. Cleft lip (Figure 11-5 G)

1. **Cleft lip occurs when:**
   a. The maxillary prominence fails to fuse with the medial nasal prominence
   b. The underlying somitomeric mesoderm and neural crest fail to expand, resulting in a **persistent labial groove**

2. Cleft lip may occur unilaterally or bilaterally. **Unilateral cleft lip** is the most common congenital malformation of the head and neck.

3. **Cleft lip and cleft palate are distinct malformations** based on their embryologic formation, even though they often occur together.

12

Nervous System

I. NEURULATION (Figure 12-1) refers to the formation and closure of the neural tube. **BMP-4** (bone morphogenetic protein), **noggin** (an inductor protein), **chordin** (an inductor protein), **FGF-8** (fibroblast growth factor), and **N-CAM** (neural cell adhesion molecule) appear to play a role in neural tube formation. The events of neurulation occur as follows:

   A. The **notochord** induces the overlying ectoderm to differentiate into **neuroectoderm** and form the **neural plate.** The notochord forms the **nucleus pulposus** of the intervertebral disk in the adult.

   B. The neural plate folds to give rise to the **neural tube,** which is open at both ends at the **anterior** and **posterior neuropores.** The anterior and posterior neuropores connect the lumen of the neural tube with the amniotic cavity.

      1. The **anterior neuropore** closes during week 4 (day 25) and becomes the **lamina terminalis.** Failure of the anterior neuropore to close results in upper neural tube defects (NTDs; e.g., **anencephaly**).

      2. The **posterior neuropore** closes during week 4 (day 27). Failure of the posterior neuropore to close results in lower NTDs (e.g., **spina bifida with myeloschisis**).

      3. NTDs can be diagnosed prenatally by detecting elevated levels of **α-fetoprotein** in the amniotic fluid. About **75% of all NTDs can be prevented** if all women capable of becoming pregnant consume **folic acid** (dose: 0.4 mg of folic acid/day).

   C. As the neural plate folds, some cells differentiate into **neural crest cells.**

   D. The rostral part of the neural tube becomes the adult **brain.**

   E. The caudal part of the neural tube becomes the adult **spinal cord.**

   F. The lumen of the neural tube gives rise to the **ventricular system** of the brain and **central canal** of the spinal cord.

II. FORMATION OF NEURAL TUBE VESICLES (Figure 12-2 and Table 12-1)

   A. During week 4, the rostral part of the neural tube forms **three primary vesicles:** the **prosencephalon** (forebrain), **mesencephalon** (midbrain), and **rhombencephalon** (hindbrain).

   B. **FGF-8, Wnt-1, En-1, En-2, and Otx-2** appear to play a role in the fundamental patterning of the mesencephalon.

   C. The **Hox complex** and **Krox-20** appear to play a role in the fundamental patterning of the rhombencephalon.

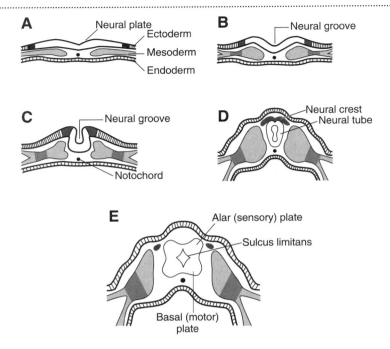

Figure 12-1. (A–E) Transverse sections of embryos at various stages showing the formation of the neural tube and neural crest cells. (E) The sulcus limitans is a groove in the lumen of the neural tube and is an important anatomic landmark, because it separates the alar (sensory) plate from the basal (motor) plate.

    D. During week 6, **five secondary vesicles** become apparent: **telencephalon, diencephalon, mesencephalon, metencephalon,** and **myelencephalon.**

III. HISTOGENESIS

    A. Neuroblasts arise from neuroectoderm and form all the neurons within the central nervous system (CNS).

    B. Glioblasts arise from neuroectoderm and form the supporting cells of the CNS. These supporting cells include:

        1. Astrocytes, which contain **glial fibrillary acidic protein (GFAP).** Astrocytes surround blood capillaries with their vascular feet.

        2. Radial glial cells, which are of astrocytic lineage and are GFAP-positive. They provide guidance for migrating neuroblasts.

        3. Oligodendrocytes, which produce the **myelin** of the CNS.

        4. Ependymocytes, which line the ventricles and the central canal.

        5. Tanycytes, which are located in the wall of the third ventricle. Tanycytes transport substances from the cerebrospinal fluid (CSF) to the hypophyseal portal system.

        6. Choroid plexus cells, which produce **CSF.** These cells are bound together by tight junctions that represent the blood-CSF barrier.

A   **B**

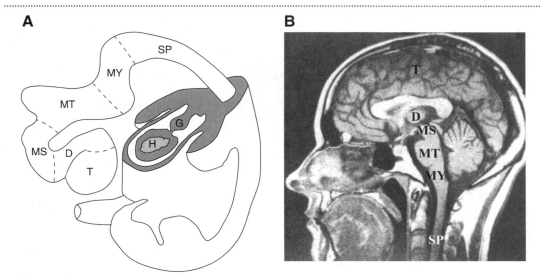

Figure 12-2.   Neural tube vesicles. (*A*) Diagram of an embryo at week 6 cross-sectioned at the level of the heart tube (*H*) and gut tube (*G*), showing the five secondary vesicles extending out from the embryo. (*B*) This median magnetic resonance (MR) image of an adult shows the derivatives of the secondary vesicles. *T* = telencephalon; *D* = diencephalon; *MS* = mesencephalon; *MT* = metencephalon; *MY* = myelencephalon; *SP* = spinal cord. (*B*, From Fleckenstein P and Tranum-Jensen J: *Anatomy in Diagnostic Imaging.* Philadelphia, WB Saunders, 1996, p 169. Copyright 1993 by Munksgaard, Copenhagen, Denmark.)

    C. Microglia (Hortega cells) arise from monocytes within the bone marrow and migrate into the CNS along with the vasculature. These cells are the macrophages of the CNS.

IV. POSITIONAL CHANGES OF THE SPINAL CORD (Figure 12-3)

    A. At week 8, the spinal cord extends the entire length of the vertebral canal as spinal nerves exit the intervertebral foramina near their level of origin. This condition does not persist owing to the disproportionate growth of the vertebral column during the fetal period.

Table 12-1
Neural Tube Vesicles and Their Adult Derivatives

Primary Vesicles	Secondary Vesicles	Adult Derivatives
Prosencephalon	Telencephalon	Cerebral hemispheres, caudate, putamen, amygdaloid, claustrum, lamina terminalis, olfactory bulbs, hippocampus
	Diencephalon	Epithalamus, subthalamus, thalamus, hypothalamus, mamillary bodies, neurohypophysis, pineal gland, globus pallidus, retina, iris, ciliary body, optic nerve (CNII), optic chiasm, optic tract
Mesencephalon	Mesencephalon	Midbrain
Rhombencephalon	Metencephalon	Pons, cerebellum
	Mylencephalon	Medulla

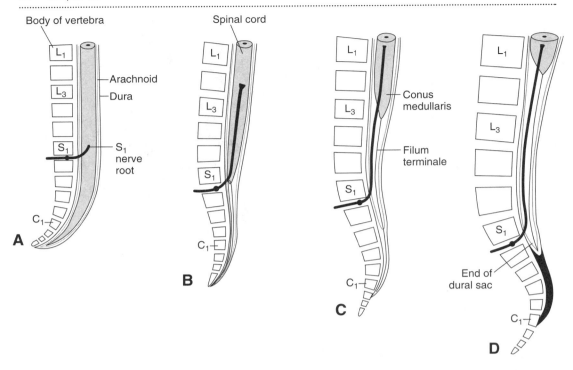

Figure 12-3. The end of the spinal cord (conus medullaris) is shown in relation to the vertebral column and meninges. (*A*) Week 8. (*B*) Week 24. (*C*) Newborn. (*D*) Adult. As the vertebral column grows, nerve roots (especially those of the lumbar and sacral segments) are elongated to form the cauda equina. The S1 nerve root is shown as an example. (Modified from Moore KL and Persaud TVN: *The Developing Human*, 6th ed. Philadelphia, WB Saunders, 1998, p 459.)

    B. At birth, the end of the spinal cord (**conus medullaris**) extends to the **L3** vertebral level.

    C. In adults, the end of the spinal cord (**conus medullaris**) extends to the **L1-L2 interspace.**

    D. The collection of dorsal and ventral nerve roots that descend below the conus medullaris is called the **cauda equina.**

    E. An extension of the pia mater forms the **filum terminale,** which anchors the spinal cord to the coccyx.

V. MENINGES

    A. The **dura mater** arises from mesoderm that surrounds the neural tube.

    B. The **pia mater** and **arachnoid** arise from neural crest cells.

VI. HYPOPHYSIS (Figure 12-4)

    A. Adenohypophysis

        1. Formation

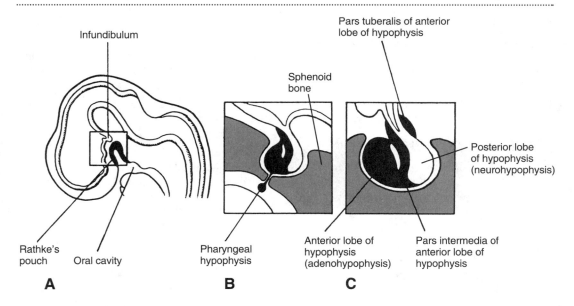

Figure 12-4. Schematic drawings illustrating the development of the hypophysis (pituitary gland). (A) A mid-sagittal section through the 6-week-old embryo, showing Rathke's pouch as a dorsal outpocketing of the oral cavity and the infundibulum as a thickening in the floor of the hypothalamus. (B, C) Development at 11 weeks and 16 weeks, respectively. The anterior lobe, the pars tuberalis, and the pars intermedia are derived from Rathke's pouch. (Modified from Sadler TW: *Langman's Medical Embryology*, 6th ed. Baltimore, Williams & Wilkins, 1990, p 373.)

    a. The adenohypophysis develops from an evagination of ectoderm lining the roof of the primitive mouth called **Rathke's pouch.**

    b. Rpx, Lhx-3, and Lhx-4 (homeobox genes) appear to play a role in the formation of Rathke's pouch.

  2. Clinical correlations

    a. **Craniopharyngioma** is a congenital cystic tumor resulting from remnants of Rathke's pouch.

    b. **Pituitary dwarfism.** A well-characterized subset of individuals with pituitary dwarfism is deficient not only in growth hormone (GH) but also in thyroid-stimulating hormone (TSH) and prolactin (PRL). The combined deficiency of GH, TSH, and PRL is caused by a genetic mutation in the **Pit-1 gene,** which encodes for a transcription factor called **Pit-1.** Pit-1 transcription factor is required for the normal transcription of GH, TSH, and PRL.

 B. **Neurohypophysis.** The neurohypophysis develops from an evagination of neuroectoderm from the **diencephalon** (i.e., specifically from the **hypothalamus**).

VII. AUTONOMIC NERVOUS SYSTEM

  A. Sympathetic system

    1. Preganglionic sympathetic neurons within the intermediolateral cell column originate from the basal plate of the neural tube (i.e., neuroectoderm).

    2. Postganglionic sympathetic neurons within the sympathetic chain ganglia and prevertebral ganglia (e.g., celiac ganglion) originate from neural crest cells.

B. Parasympathetic system

    1. Preganglionic parasympathetic neurons within the nuclei of the midbrain (CN III), pons (CN VII), medulla (CN IX and CN X), and spinal cord at S2-S4 originate from the basal plate of the neural tube (i.e., neuroectoderm).

    2. Postganglionic parasympathetic neurons within the ciliary (CN III), pterygopalatine (CN VII), submandibular (CN VII), otic (CN IX), enteric (CN X), and abdominal/pelvic cavity ganglia originate from neural crest cells.

VIII. CLINICAL CORRELATIONS

    A. Variations of spina bifida and encephalocele (Figure 12-5). Spina bifida occurs when the bony vertebral arches fail to form properly, creating a **vertebral defect,** usually in the **sacrolumbar** region. Encephalocele occurs when the bony skull fails to form properly, creating a **skull defect,** usually in the **occipital** region.

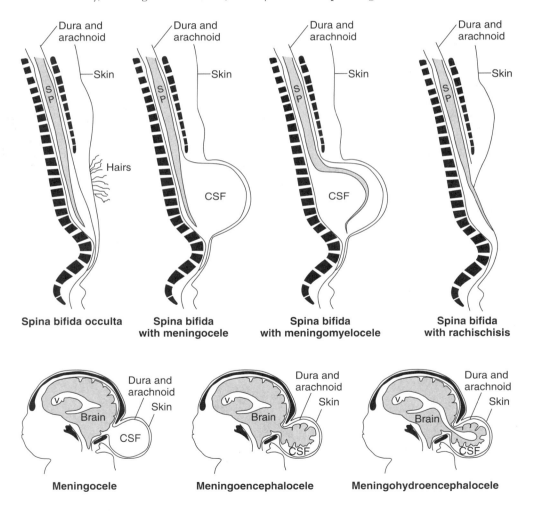

Figure 12-5. Variations of spina bifida and encephalocele. *SP* = spinal cord; *CSF* = cerebrospinal fluid; *V* = ventricle. (Modified from Haines DE [ed]: *Fundamental Neuroscience.* New York, Churchill Livingstone, 1997, p 69.)

1. **Spina bifida occulta (Figure 12-6 A)** is evidenced by a **tuft of hair** in the sacrolumbar region. It is the least severe variation and occurs in 10% of the population.

2. **Spina bifida with meningocele** occurs when the meninges project through a vertebral defect and form a sac filled with CSF. The spinal cord remains in its normal position.

3. **Spina bifida with meningomyelocele (Figure 12-6 B).** This form occurs when the meninges and spinal cord project through a vertebral defect to form a sac.

4. **Spina bifida with rachischisis (Figure 12-6 C)** occurs when the posterior neuropore fails to close, thus creating an **open neural tube** that lies on the surface of the back. It is **the most severe type** of spina bifida, causing paralysis from the level of the defect caudally.

5. **Meningocele (Figure 12-6 D)** occurs when the meninges project through the skull defect. It is a rare condition.

6. **Meningoencephalocele** occurs when the meninges and brain protrude through the skull defect. This defect usually comes to medical attention within the infant's first few days or weeks of life. The outcome is poor (i.e., approximately 75% of the infants die or are severely retarded).

7. **Meningohydroencephalocele (Figure 12-6 E)** occurs when the meninges, brain, and a portion of the ventricle protrude through the skull defect.

B. **Anencephaly (meroanencephaly) (see Figure 12-6 F, G)** occurs when the anterior neuropore fails to close. It results in failure of the brain to develop (however, a rudimentary brain stem is present), failure of the lamina terminalis to form, and failure of the bony cranial vault to form.

   1. Anencephaly is **incompatible with extrauterine life.** If not stillborn, infants with anencephaly survive for only a few hours or few weeks. Anencephaly is the most common serious birth defect seen in stillborn infants.

   2. Anencephaly is **easily diagnosed by ultrasound,** and a therapeutic abortion is usually performed at the mother's request.

C. **Arnold-Chiari malformation (Figure 12-7 A)** occurs when vermis and tonsils of the cerebellum and medulla oblongata herniate through the foramen magnum.

   1. **Clinical signs** are caused by compression of the medulla oblongata and stretching of CN IX, CN X, and CN XII. They include spastic dysphonia, difficulty in swallowing, laryngeal stridor (vibrating sound heard during respiration as a result of obstructed airways), diminished gag reflex, apnea, and vocal cord paralysis.

   2. This malformation is commonly associated with a **lumbar meningomyelocele, platybasia** (bone malformation of base of skull) along with malformation of the occipitovertebral joint, and **hydrocephalus** (caused by several factors; however, approximately 50% of cases demonstrate **aqueductal stenosis**).

D. **Hydrocephalus** is a dilatation of the ventricles caused by an excess of CSF, which may result from either a blockage of CSF circulation or rarely an overproduction of CSF (e.g., due to a choroid plexus papilloma).

   1. **Communicating (nonobstructive) hydrocephalus.** In this type of hydrocephalus there is free communication between the ventricles and the subarachnoid space. The blockage of CSF in this type of hydrocephalus is usually in the subarachnoid space or arachnoid granulations and results in the enlargement of all the ventricular cavities as well as the subarachnoid space.

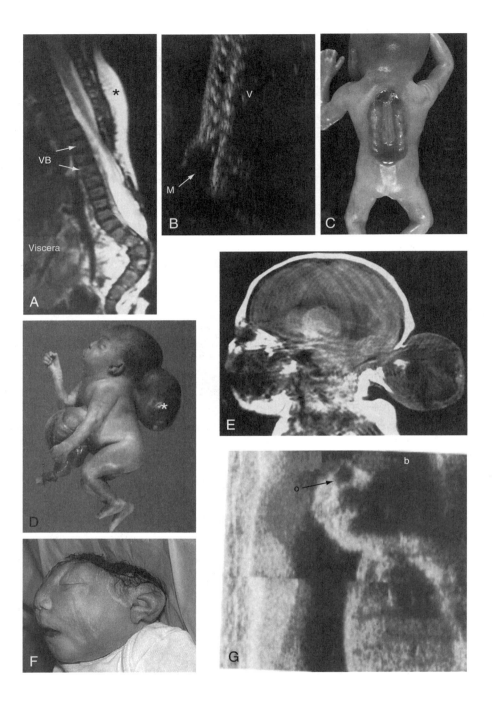

Figure 12-6. (A) **Spina bifida occulta.** Note the presence of the bony vertebral bodies (*VB*) along the entire length of the vertebral column. However, the bony spinous processes terminate much higher (*) because the vertebral arches fail to form properly. This creates a vertebral defect. The spinal cord is intact. (B) **Spina bifida with meningomyelocele** as seen on an ultrasonogram of a 14-week-old fetus. Note the cyst-like protrusion (*m* = meningomyelocele) and the normal vertebrae (*v*) superior to the meningomyelocele. (C) **Spina bifida with rachischisis** in a newborn infant. Note the open neural tube. (D) Photograph of an **occipital meningocele** (*) in a fetus. (E) **Meningohydroencephalocele** as seen on magnetic resonance image (MRI). (F) **Anencephaly** in newborn infant. (G) **Anencephaly as seen on an ultrasonogram** of a 14-week-old fetus. Note the orbit (*o*) and the remnant of brain (*b*). (A and E, from Haines DE [ed]: *Fundamental Neuroscience*. New York, Churchill Livingstone, 1997, pp 68, 69. B and G, Courtesy of Dr. Lyndon M. Hill, Magee-Women's Hospital, Pittsburgh, PA. From Moore KL and Persaud TVN: *The Developing Human*, 6th ed. Philadelphia, WB Saunders, 1998, p 464, 480. C, From Papp Z [ed]: *Atlas of Fetal Diagnosis*. Amsterdam, Elsevier, 1992, p 128. D, From Carlson BM: *Human Embryology and Developmental Biology*, 2nd ed. St. Louis, CV Mosby, 1999, p 244.)

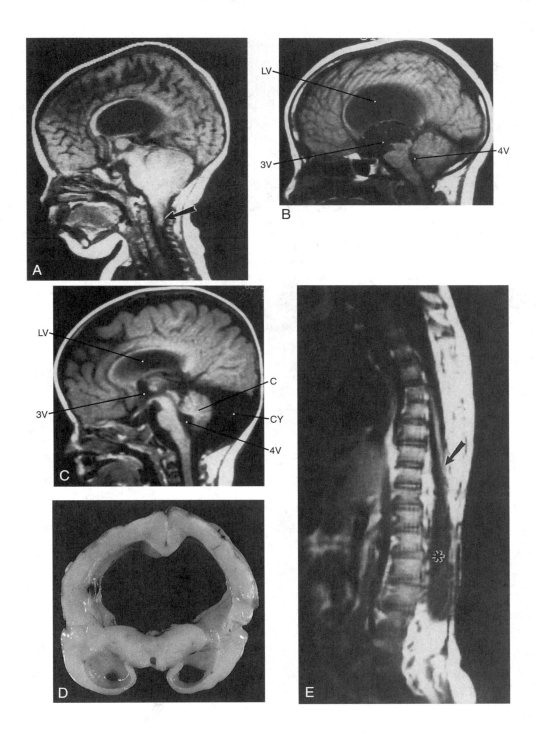

Figure 12-7. (A) **Arnold-Chiari malformation** as seen on a magnetic resonance image (MRI). Note the herniation of the brain stem and cerebellum (*arrow*) through the foramen magnum. (B) **Congenital aqueductal stenosis** as seen on an MRI. Note the selective enlargement of the lateral ventricle (LV) and third ventricle (3V). The fourth ventricle (4V) is normal in size. (C) **Dandy-Walker syndrome** as seen on MRI. *LV* = lateral ventricle; *3V* = third ventricle; *C* = cerebellar vermis; *CY* = cyst; *4V* = fourth ventricle. (D) **Holoprosencephaly.** Note the fuse thalami at the base of the one large ventricle. (E) A **tethered spinal cord** as seen on MRI. Note the tethered spinal cord (*arrow*) and a dilated thecal sac (***) along with a posterior bone defect. (A and E, from Heimer L: *The Human Brain and Spinal Cord: Functional Neuroanatomy and Dissection Guide,* 2nd ed. New York, Springer-Verlag, 1995, p 39. B and C, from Afifi AK, Bergman RA: *Functional Neuroanatomy: Text and Atlas.* New York, McGraw-Hill, 1998, pp 580 and 585. D, From Papp Z [ed]: *Atlas of Fetal Diagnosis.* Amsterdam, Elsevier, 1992, p 101.)

2. Noncommunicating (obstructive) hydrocephalus. In this type of hydrocephalus there is a lack of communication between the ventricles and the subarachnoid space. The blockage of CSF in this type of hydrocephalus is in the foramen of Monro, cerebral aqueduct, or foramina of Magendie and Luschka and results in the enlargement of only those ventricular cavities proximal to the blockage. There are **two types of congenital hydrocephalus,** both of which produce a noncommunicating (obstructive) hydrocephalus:

  a. Congenital aqueductal stenosis (Figure 12-7 B) is **the most common cause** of congenital hydrocephalus. This type may be transmitted by an X-linked trait, or it may be caused by cytomegalovirus or toxoplasmosis.

  b. Dandy-Walker syndrome (see Figure 12-7 C) appears to be associated with **atresia of the outlet foramina of Luschka and Magendie,** although this remains controversial. This syndrome is usually associated with dilatation of the fourth ventricle, agenesis of the cerebellar vermis, occipital meningocele, and frequently agenesis of the splenium of the corpus callosum.

E. Holoprosencephaly (arhinencephaly) (Figure 12-7 D) occurs when the prosencephalon fails to cleave down the midline such that the telencephalon contains a single ventricular cavity.

  1. Holoprosencephaly is characterized by the **absence of olfactory bulbs and tracts** (arhinencephaly).

  2. Holoprosencephaly is **often seen in trisomy 13** (Patau's syndrome).

  3. This is the most severe manifestation of **fetal alcohol syndrome,** resulting from alcohol abuse during pregnancy (especially in the first 4 weeks of pregnancy).

F. Tethered spinal cord (Figure 12-7 E) occurs when a thick and short filum terminale forms. The result is weakness and sensory deficits in the lower extremity and also a neurogenic bladder. Tethered spinal cord is frequently associated with lipomatous tumors or lipomyelomeningoceles. Deficits usually improve after transection.

G. Chordoma is a tumor that arises from remnants of the notochord.

13

Ear

I. OVERVIEW. The ear is the organ of **balance** and **hearing.** It consists of an **internal,** a **middle,** and an **external ear.**

II. INTERNAL EAR (Figure 13-1). The internal ear develops in Week 4 from a thickening of the **surface ectoderm** called the **otic placode.**

    A. Otic vesicle. The otic placode invaginates into the mesoderm adjacent to the rhombencephalon and becomes the otic vesicle. The otic vesicle divides into utricular and saccular portions.

        1. Utricular portion. This portion of the otic vesicle gives rise to:
            a. The **utricle,** which contains the sensory hair cells and otoliths of the macula utriculi. It responds to linear acceleration and the force of gravity.
            b. The **semicircular ducts,** contain the sensory hair cells of the cristae ampullaris. They respond to angular acceleration.
            c. The **vestibular ganglion of cranial nerve (CN) VIII,** which lies at the base of the internal auditory meatus.
            d. The **endolymphatic duct and sac,** a membranous canal connects with the saccule and utricle and terminates in a blind dilatation beneath the dura. The endolymphatic sac absorbs endolymph.

        2. Saccular portion. This portion of the otic vesicle gives rise to:
            a. The **saccule,** which contains the sensory hair cells and otoliths of the macula sacculi. It responds to linear acceleration and the force of gravity.
            b. The **cochlear duct (organ of Corti).** This duct has pitch (tonotopic) localization whereby high frequencies (20,000 Hz) are detected at the base and low frequencies (20 Hz) are detected at the apex.
            c. The **spiral ganglion of CN VIII,** which lies in the modiolus of the bony labyrinth.

    B. Membranous labyrinth and bony labyrinth

        1. The membranous labyrinth consists of all the structures derived from the otic vesicle **(Table 13-1).**

        2. The membranous labyrinth is initially surrounded by mesoderm, which later becomes cartilaginous and ossifies to become the **bony labyrinth** of the temporal bone.

        3. The mesoderm closest to the membranous labyrinth degenerates, thus forming the **perilymphatic space** that contains **perilymph.**

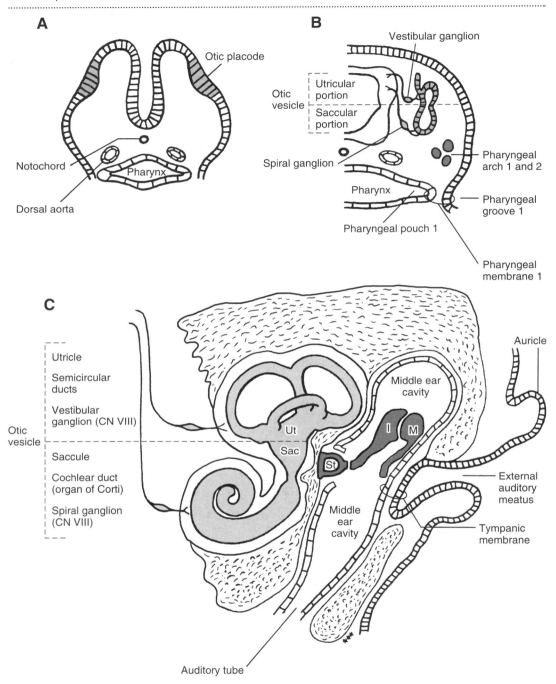

Figure 13-1.   Schematic transverse sections show the formation of the otic placode and otic vesicle from the surface ectoderm. (*A*) The otic placode invaginates into the mesoderm and becomes the otic vesicle. The mesoderm later develops into bone, that is, the bony labyrinth. (*B*) The vestibular and spiral ganglia of CN VIII are derived from the otic vesicle. (*C*) The adult ear. M = malleus; I = incus; St = stapes; Ut = utricle; Sac = saccule. (From Dudek RW, Fix JD: *BRS Embryology,* 2nd ed. Baltimore, Williams & Wilkins, 1998, p 106.)

Table 13-1

Derivation of the Structures of the Ear

Embryonic Structure	Adult Derivative
	Internal Ear
Otic Vesicle	
Utricular portion	Utricle, semicircular ducts, vestibular ganglion of CN VIII, endolymphatic duct and sac
Saccular portion	Saccule, cochlear duct (organ of Corti), spiral ganglion of CN VIII
	Middle Ear
Pharyngeal arch 1	Malleus, incus, tensor tympani muscle
Pharyngeal arch 2	Stapes, stapedius muscle
Pharyngeal pouch 1	Auditory tube and middle ear cavity
Pharyngeal membrane 1	Tympanic membrane
	External Ear
Pharyngeal groove 1	External auditory meatus
Auricular hillocks	Auricle

CN = cranial nerve.

4. The membranous labyrinth is suspended within the bony labyrinth by perilymph. Perilymph, which is similar in composition to **cerebrospinal fluid,** communicates with the subarachnoid space via the **perilymphatic duct.**

III. MIDDLE EAR (Figure 13-1)

A. Ossicles. The ossicles include the malleus, the incus, and the stapes.

1. **Malleus.** The malleus develops from the cartilage of **pharyngeal arch 1** (Meckel's cartilage). It is attached to the tympanic membrane and is moved by the **tensor tympani muscle,** which is innervated by CN V-3.

2. Incus. The incus develops from the cartilage of **pharyngeal arch 1** (Meckel's cartilage). It articulates with the malleus and stapes.

3. **Stapes.** The stapes develops from the cartilage of **pharyngeal arch 2** (Reichert's cartilage). The stapes is moved by the **stapedius muscle,** which is innervated by CN VII. It is attached to the oval window of the vestibule.

B. Auditory tube and middle ear cavity. These develop from **pharyngeal pouch 1.**

C. Tympanic membrane. This membrane develops from **pharyngeal membrane 1.** It separates the middle ear from the external auditory meatus of the external ear; it is innervated by CN V-3 and CN IX.

IV. EXTERNAL EAR (Figure 13-1)

A. External auditory meatus. The external auditory meatus develops from **pharyngeal groove 1.** It becomes filled with ectodermal cells, forming a temporary **meatal plug** that disappears before birth. The external auditory meatus is innervated by **CN V-3 and CN IX.**

B. Auricle. The auricle develops from **six auricular hillocks** that surround pharyngeal groove 1. It is innervated by **CN V-3, CN VII, CN IX, and CN X** and also by cervical nerves C2 and C3.

V. CLINICAL CORRELATIONS

A. Congenital deafness. The organ of Corti may be damaged by exposure to **rubella virus,** especially during weeks 7 and 8 of development.

B. Malformation of the auricles in chromosomal syndromes. This occurs in **Down syndrome** (trisomy 21), **Patau's syndrome** (trisomy 13), and **Edward's syndrome** (trisomy 18).

C. Atresia of the external auditory meatus results from failure of the meatal plug to canalize; this results in conduction deafness and is usually associated with first arch syndrome.

D. Congenital cholesteatoma (epidermoid cyst) is a frequent cause of conduction deafness. This cyst is a benign tumor that is found in the middle ear cavity; it is thought to develop from "epidermoid thickenings" of endodermal lining cells.

14
Eye

I. DEVELOPMENT OF THE OPTIC VESICLE (Figure 14-1). The optic vesicle begins to develop at day 22 with the formation of the **optic sulcus.** The optic sulcus evaginates from the wall of the diencephalon as the **optic vesicle,** consisting of **neuroectoderm.** The optic vesicle invaginates and forms a double-layered **optic cup** and **optic stalk.**

   A. The optic cup and its derivatives (Table 14-1). The double-layered optic cup consists of an **outer pigment layer** and an **inner neural layer.**

      1. Retina
         a. The **outer pigment layer of the optic cup** gives rise to the **pigment layer of the retina.**
         b. The **intraretinal space** separates the pigment layer of the retina from the neural layer of the retina. Although the intraretinal space is obliterated in the adult, it remains a weakened area prone to retinal detachment.
         c. The **inner neural layer of the optic cup** gives rise to the neural layer of the retina (i.e., the rods and cones, bipolar cells, and the ganglion cells).

      2. Iris (Figure 14-2)
         a. The epithelium of the iris develops from the anterior portions of both the outer pigment layer and the inner neural layer of the optic cup, which explains its histologic appearance of two layers of columnar epithelium.
         b. The stroma of the iris develops from mesoderm continuous with the choroid.
         c. The iris contains the **dilator pupillae muscle** and the **sphincter pupillae muscle,** which are formed from the epithelium of the outer pigment layer by a transformation of these epithelial cells into contractile cells.

      3. Ciliary body (see Figure 14-2)
         a. The epithelium of the ciliary body develops from the anterior portions of both the outer pigment layer and the inner neural layer of the optic cup, which explains its histologic appearance of two layers of columnar epithelium.
         b. The stroma of the ciliary body develops from mesoderm continuous with the choroid.
         c. The ciliary body contains the **ciliary muscle,** which is formed from mesoderm within the choroid.
         d. Ciliary processes are components of the ciliary body.
            (1) The ciliary processes produce **aqueous humor,** which circulates through the posterior and anterior chambers and drains into the venous circulation via the **trabecular meshwork** and the **canal of Schlemm.**
            (2) The ciliary processes give rise to the **suspensory fibers** of the lens (ciliary zonule), which suspend the lens.

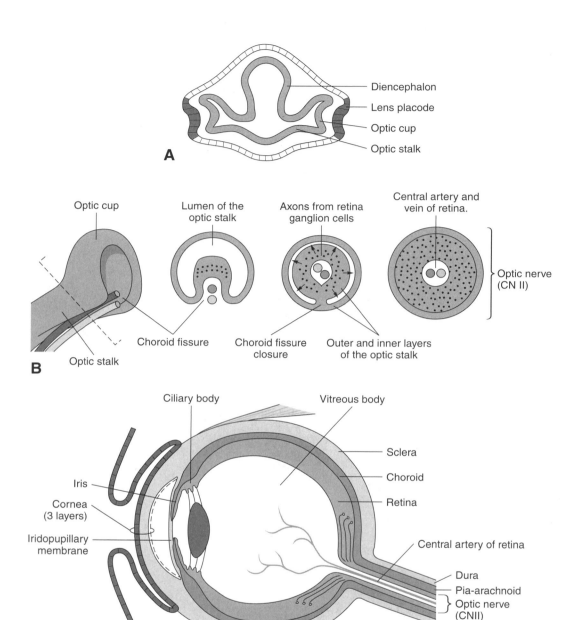

Figure 14-1. (A) The optic cup and optic stalk are evaginations of the diencephalon. The optic cup induces surface ectoderm to differentiate into the lens placode. (B) Formation of the optic nerve (CN II) from the optic stalk. The choroid fissure, which is located on the undersurface of the optic stalk, permits access of the hyaloid artery and vein to the inner aspect of the eye. The choroid fissure eventually closes. As ganglion cells form in the retina, axons accumulate in the optic stalk and cause the inner and outer layers of the optic stalk to fuse, obliterating the lumen (or intraretinal space) and forming the optic nerve. (C) The adult eye. Note that the sclera is continuous with the dura mater and the choroid is continuous with the pia-arachnoid. The iridopupillary membrane is normally obliterated. (Adapted from Dudek RW, Fix JD: *BRS Embryology,* 2nd ed. Baltimore, Williams & Wilkins, 1998, p 114.)

Table 14-1

Embryonic Eye Structures and Their Adult Derivatives

Embryonic Structure	Adult Derivative
Diencephalon (neuroectoderm)	
Optic cup	Retina, iris epithelium, dilator and sphincter pupillae muscles of the iris, ciliary body epithelium
Optic stalk	Optic nerve (CN II), optic chiasm, optic tract
Surface ectoderm	Lens, anterior epithelium of the cornea
Mesoderm	Sclera, choroid, stroma of the iris, stroma of the ciliary body, ciliary muscle, substantia propria of the cornea, corneal endothelium, vitreous body, central artery and vein of the retina, extraocular muscles

B. The optic stalk and its derivatives

    1. The optic stalk contains the **choroid fissure** in which the **hyaloid vessels** are found. These vessels later become the **central artery and vein of the retina.** The optic stalk contains axons from the ganglion cell layer.

    2. The choroid fissure closes during week 7 so that the optic stalk, together with the axons of the ganglion cells, forms the **optic nerve (CN II), optic chiasm, and optic tract.**

    3. The **optic nerve (CN II)** is a tract of the diencephalon.
        a. The optic nerve is not completely myelinated until 3 months after birth; it is myelinated by oligodendrocytes.
        b. This nerve is not capable of regeneration after transection.
        c. It is invested by the meninges and, therefore, is surrounded by a subarachnoid space (papilledema).

II. DEVELOPMENT OF OTHER EYE STRUCTURES (see Table 14-1)

    A. Sclera. The sclera develops from mesoderm surrounding the optic cup. It forms an **outer fibrous layer** that is continuous with the dura mater posteriorly and the cornea anteriorly.

    B. Choroid. The choroid develops from mesoderm surrounding the optic cup. It forms a vascular layer which is continuous with the pia/arachnoid posteriorly and the iris/ciliary body anteriorly.

    C. Anterior chamber. This chamber develops from mesoderm over the anterior aspect of the eye, which is continuous with the sclera and undergoes vacuolization to form a chamber. The anterior chamber essentially splits the mesoderm into two layers:

        1. The mesoderm posterior to the anterior chamber is called the **iridopupillary membrane,** which is normally resorbed before birth.

        2. The mesoderm anterior to the anterior chamber develops into the **substantia propria of the cornea** and the **corneal endothelium.**

    D. Cornea. The cornea develops from both surface ectoderm and mesoderm lying anterior to the anterior chamber. The surface ectoderm forms the **anterior epithelium of the cornea.** The mesoderm forms the **substantia propria of the cornea** and **corneal endothelium.**

    E. Lens. The lens develops from surface ectoderm, which forms the **lens placode.** The

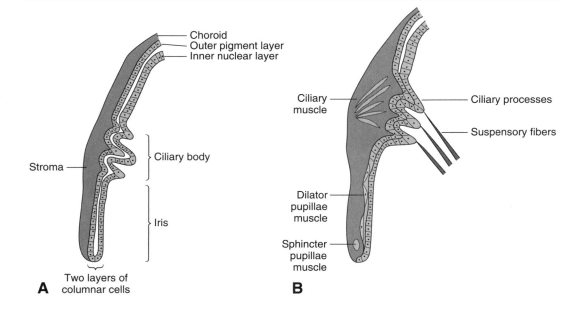

Figure 14-2.   (A, B) Sagittal sections through the developing iris and ciliary body. The iris and ciliary body form from the outer pigment layer and inner neural layer of the optic cup. In the adult, this embryologic origin is reflected histologically by two layers of columnar epithelium that line both the iris and the ciliary body. (Adapted from Dudek RW, Fix JD: *BRS Embryology*, 2nd ed. Baltimore, Williams & Wilkins, 1998, p 116.)

lens placode invaginates to form the **lens vesicle.** The cells of the posterior wall of the lens vesicle elongate, lose their nuclei, and form the lens fibers of the adult lens.

F. **Vitreous body.** The vitreous body develops from mesoderm that migrates through the choroid fissure and forms a transparent gelatinous substance between the lens and the retina. It contains the **hyaloid artery,** which later obliterates to form the **hyaloid canal** of the adult eye.

G. **Canal of Schlemm.** The canal of Schlemm is found at the sclerocorneal junction called the **limbus.** This canal drains the aqueous humor into the venous circulation. Obstruction results in increased intraocular pressure (**glaucoma**).

H. **Extraocular muscles.** These muscles develop from mesoderm surrounding the optic cup that has been called **preotic myotomes,** although in humans the origin is still controversial.

III. CLINICAL CORRELATIONS

A. **Coloboma iridis (Figure 14-3A)** is a cleft in the iris caused by failure of the choroid fissure to close in week 7 of development. This cleft may extend into the ciliary body, retina, choroid, or optic nerve. Palpebral coloboma, a notch in the eyelid, results from a defect in the developing eyelid.

B. **Congenital cataracts (see Figure 14-3B)** are opacities of the lens and are usually bilateral. They are common and may result from rubella virus infection, toxoplasmosis, congenital syphilis, Down syndrome (trisomy 21), or galactosemia (an inborn error of metabolism).

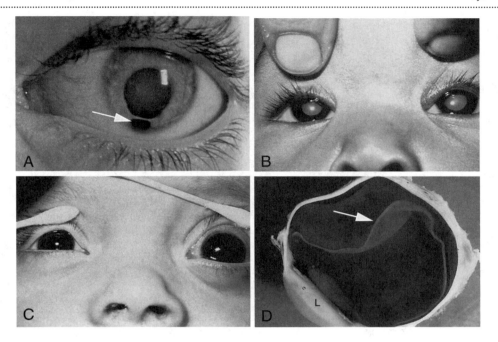

Figure 14-3. (A) Coloboma iridis. Note the cleft in the iris (*black spot at arrow*). (B) Congenital cataracts. Note the lens opacities in both eyes. (C) Congenital glaucoma (buphthalmos). Note the enlarged left eye and the normal right eye. (D) Detached retina. Note the retina (*arrow*) detached from the choroid and sclera. L = lens. (A, From Bergsma D [ed]: *Birth Defects: Atlas and Compendium.* Baltimore, Williams & Wilkins, 1973, Fig. 6.47. B–D, From Gilbert-Barness E: *Potter's Atlas of Fetal and Infant Pathology.* St Louis, CV Mosby, 1998, pp 366 and 370.)

    C. **Congenital glaucoma (buphthalmos; see Figure 14-3C)** is increased intraocular pressure due to abnormal development of the canal of Schlemm or the iridocorneal filtration angle. It is usually genetically determined, but it may result from maternal rubella infection.

    D. **Detached retina (see Figure 14-3D)** may be caused by head trauma or it may be congenital. The site of detachment is between the outer and inner layers of the optic cup (i.e., between the retinal pigment epithelial layer and the layer of rods and cones of the neural retina).

    E. **Persistent iridopupillary membrane** consists of strands of connective tissue that partially cover the pupil; this membrane seldom affects vision.

    F. **Microphthalmia** is a small eye, usually associated with intrauterine infections from the TORCH (toxoplasma, rubella virus, cytomegalovirus, and herpes simplex virus) group of microorganisms.

    G. **Anophthalmia** is absence of the eye. This condition is caused by failure of the optic vesicle to form.

    H. **Cyclopia** involves a single orbit and one eye. It is caused by failure of median cerebral structures to develop.

I. **Retinocele** results from herniation of the retina into the sclera or failure of the choroid fissure to close.

J. **Retrolental fibroplasia** (retinopathy of prematurity) is an oxygen-induced retinopathy seen in premature infants.

K. **Papilledema** is edema of the optic disk (papilla) due to increased intracranial pressure. This pressure is reflected into the subarachnoid space, which surrounds the optic nerve (CN II).

L. **Retinitis pigmentosa (RP)** is hereditary degeneration and atrophy of the retina.

    1. RP may be transmitted as an autosomal recessive, autosomal dominant, or X-linked trait.

    2. RP may be caused by abetalipoproteinemia (Bassen-Kornzweig syndrome); progression of this disease may be arrested with massive doses of vitamin A.

    3. RP is characterized by a degeneration of the rods, night blindness (nyctalopia), and "gun barrel vision."

M. **Retinoblastoma (RB)** is a retinal tumor that occurs in childhood and develops from precursor cells in the immature retina:

    1. The RB gene is located on chromosome 13 and encodes for RB protein, which binds to a gene regulatory protein and causes suppression of the cell cycle. Thus, the RB gene is a **tumor-suppressor gene** (also called an **antioncogene**).

    2. A mutation in the RB gene will encode an abnormal RB protein such that there is no suppression of the cell cycle. This leads to the formation of RB.

    3. Hereditary RB causes multiple tumors in both eyes. Nonhereditary RB causes a tumor in one eye.

15

Body Cavities

I. FORMATION OF THE INTRAEMBRYONIC COELOM (Figure 15-1 A–C) begins when spaces coalesce within the lateral mesoderm and form a horseshoe-shaped space that opens into the chorionic cavity (extraembryonic coelom) on the right and left sides.

II. PARTITIONING OF THE INTRAEMBRYONIC COELOM. The intraembryonic coelom is initially one continuous space. In order to form the definitive adult pericardial, pleural, and peritoneal cavities, two partitions must develop: the **paired pleuropericardial membranes** and the **diaphragm.**

  A. The **paired pleuropericardial membranes (Figure 15-1D)** are sheets of somatic mesoderm that separate the pericardial cavity from the pleural cavities. They develop into the definitive **fibrous pericardium** that surrounds the adult heart.

  B. The **diaphragm (Figure 15-1E)** separates the pleural cavities from the peritoneal cavity. It is formed through the fusion of tissue from four different sources:

   1. The **septum transversum,** a thick mass of mesoderm between the primitive heart tube and the developing liver, is the primordium of the **central tendon of the diaphragm** in the adult.

   2. The **paired pleuroperitoneal membranes** are sheets of somatic mesoderm that appear to develop from the dorsal and dorsolateral body wall.

   3. The **dorsal mesentery of the esophagus** is invaded by myoblasts and forms the **crura of the diaphragm** in the adult.

   4. The **body wall** contributes muscle to the peripheral portions of the definitive diaphragm.

III. POSITIONAL CHANGES OF THE DIAPHRAGM

  A. During week 4, the developing diaphragm becomes innervated by the **phrenic nerves,** which originate from C3, C4, and C5 and pass through the pleuropericardial membranes. (This explains the definitive location of the phrenic nerves associated with the fibrous pericardium.)

  B. By week 8, there is an apparent **descent of the diaphragm to L1** because of the rapid growth of the neural tube. The phrenic nerves are carried along with the "descending diaphragm," which explains their unusually long length in the adult.

IV. CLINICAL CORRELATIONS

  A. **Esophageal hiatal hernia** is a herniation of the stomach through the esophageal hiatus into the pleural cavity, caused by an abnormally large esophageal hiatus. Esopha-

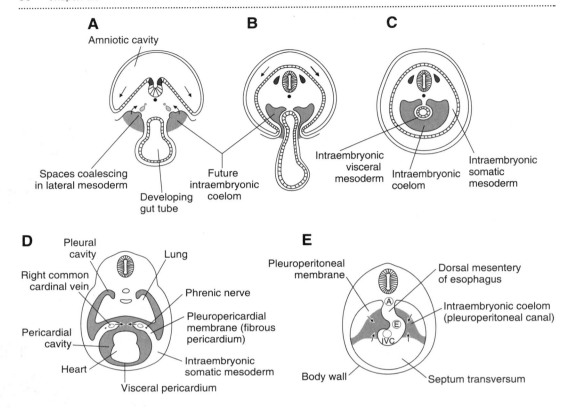

Figure 15-1. Formation and partitioning of the intraembryonic coelom (IC). (A–C) Cross-sections show various stages of IC formation while the embryo undergoes lateral folding. (D) This cross-section shows two folds of intraembryonic somatic mesoderm carrying the phrenic nerves and common cardinal veins. The two folds fuse in the midline (*arrows*) to form the pleuropericardial membrane. This separates the pericardial cavity (*shaded*) from the pleural cavity (*shaded*). (E) A cross-section of an embryo at week 5 showing the four components that fuse (*arrows*) to form the diaphragm, which closes off the intraembryonic coelom between the pleural and peritoneal cavities. The portions of the intraembryonic coelom that connect the pleural and pericardial cavities in the embryo are called the pleuroperitoneal canals (*shaded*). A = aorta; E = esophagus; IVC = inferior vena cava. (Adapted from Dudek RW, Fix JD: *BRS Embryology*, 2nd ed. Baltimore, Williams & Wilkins, 1998, pp 237–239.)

geal hiatal hernia renders the esophagogastric sphincter incompetent so that stomach contents reflux into the esophagus. The **clinical sign** in the newborn is **vomiting (frequently projectile)** when the infant is laid on its back after feeding.

B. Congenital diaphragmatic hernia (Figure 15-2) is a herniation of abdominal contents into the pleural cavity, caused by a failure of the pleuroperitoneal membrane to develop or fuse with the other components of the diaphragm. It is found most commonly on the **left posterolateral side.** The hernia is usually life threatening, because abdominal contents compress the lung buds and cause pulmonary hypoplasia. **Clinical signs** in the newborn consist of an **unusually flat abdomen, breathlessness, and cyanosis.**

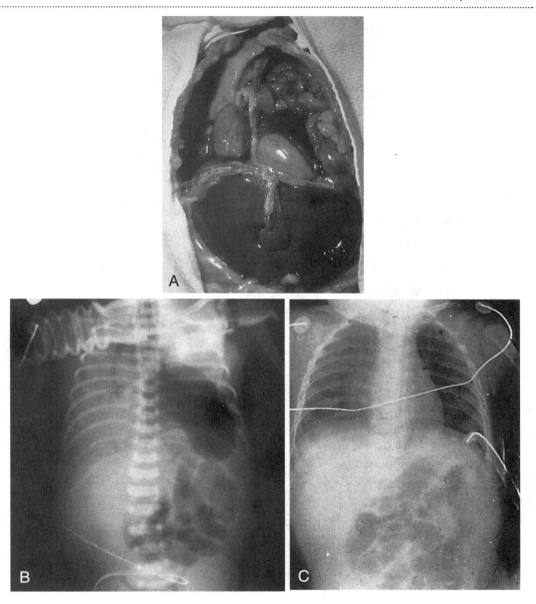

Figure 15-2. (A) A congenital diaphragmatic hernia. Note the defect in the diaphragm, which allows loops of intestine and a portion of the liver to enter the pleural cavity. There is attendant pulmonary hypoplasia. (B) Radiograph of a congenital diaphragmatic hernia. Note the loops of intestine within the pleural cavity as indicated by the bowel gas above and below the diaphragm and the mediastinal shift to the right. (C) Radiograph after surgical repair of a congenital diaphragmatic hernia. Note the bowel gas present only below the diaphragm and the mediastinal shift back to the midline. (A, From Gilbert-Barness E: *Potter's Atlas of Fetal and Infant Pathology*. St Louis, CV Mosby, 1998, p 172. B and C, from Aladjen S, Vidyasagar D: *Atlas of Perinatology*. Philadelphia, WB Saunders, 1982, pp 295, 375.)

16

Integumentary System

I. SKIN. The skin consists of two layers: the outer layer, or **epidermis,** and the deeper, connective tissue layer, or **dermis.** Skin functions as a barrier against infection, serves thermoregulation, and protects the body against dehydration.

A. Epidermis. The epidermis is derived from the ectoderm.

1. Early development
- **a.** Initially, the epidermis consists of a single layer of ectodermal cells that give rise to an overlying **periderm** layer.
- **b.** The epidermis soon becomes a **three-layered structure** consisting of the **stratum basale** (mitotically active), the **intermediate layer** (progeny of stratum basale), and the **periderm.**
- **c.** Peridermal cells are eventually desquamated; they form part of the **vernix caseosa,** a greasy substance of peridermal cells and sebum from the sebaceous glands that protects the embryo's skin.

2. Later development. The definitive adult layers are formed through the inductive influence of the dermis. The ectodermal cells give rise to five cell layers:
- **a.** Stratum basale (stratum germinativum)
- **b.** Stratum spinosum
- **c.** Stratum lucidum
- **d.** Stratum granulosum
- **e.** Stratum corneum. This layer is associated with the expression of **56.5-kda keratin, 67-kda keratin,** and **filaggrin** (a binding protein).

3. Other cells of the epidermis
- **a.** **Melanoblasts** are derived from **neural crest cells** that migrate into the stratum basal of the epidermis. These cells differentiate into melanocytes by midpregnancy, when pigment granules called **melanosomes** are observed.
- **b.** **Langerhans cells** are derived from the **bone marrow (mesoderm)** and migrate into the epidermis. These cells are involved in antigen presentation.
- **c.** **Merkel cells** are of uncertain origin. They are associated with free nerve endings and probably function as mechanoreceptors.

B. Dermis. The dermis is derived from both the somatic mesoderm, which is located just beneath the ectoderm, and mesoderm of the dermatomes of the body. It is derived from neural crest cells in the head and neck region (see Chapter 11).

1. Early development. The dermis initially consists of loosely aggregated mesodermal cells that are frequently referred to as **mesenchymal cells** (or **mesenchyme**). The mesenchymal cells secrete a watery type of extracellular matrix that is rich in glycogen and hyaluronic acid.

2. Later development

    a. Mesenchymal cells differentiate into fibroblasts, which secrete increasing amounts of collagen and elastic fibers into the extracellular matrix.

    b. Vascularization occurs.

    c. Sensory nerves grow into the dermis.

    d. The dermis forms projections into the epidermis called **dermal papillae,** which contain tactile sensory receptors (e.g., Meissner's corpuscles).

C. Clinical correlations

    1. Albinism

        a. **Oculocutaneous albinism** (classic type) is an autosomal recessive trait in which **melanocytes fail to produce melanin** in the skin, hair, and eyes. The cause is **an absence of tyrosinase activity.**

        b. **Piebaldism,** an autosomal dominant disorder, is a localized albinism in which there is a lack of melanin in isolated patches of skin or hair.

        c. Albinism predisposes to basal and squamous cell carcinoma and also to malignant melanoma.

    2. **Ichthyosis** is an X-linked disorder of keratinization characterized by dryness and scaling of the skin.

    3. **Psoriasis** is a skin disease characterized by **excessive cell proliferation** in the stratum basale and stratum spinosum, resulting in thickening of the epidermis and shorter regeneration time of the epidermis.

    4. **Ehlers-Danlos syndrome (Figure 16-1 A, B)** is characterized by extremely stretchable and fragile skin, hypermobile joints, aneurysms of blood vessels, and rupture of the bowel. It is caused by a defect of the gene for **peptidyl lysine hydroxylase,** which is an enzyme necessary for the hydroxylation of lysine residues of collagen. Type I and type III collagen are mainly affected.

    5. **Hemangiomas (Figure 16-1 C, D)** are vascular malformations, that is, benign tumors of endothelial cells. They produce "birth marks" on the skin. A **port-wine stain** is a birth mark covering the area of distribution of the trigeminal nerve (CN V) that is frequently associated with a hemangioma of the meninges called **Sturge-Weber syndrome.**

II. HAIR AND NAILS. Hair and nails are derived from the ectoderm.

A. Hair (Figure 16-2)

    1. At week 12, ectodermal cells from the stratum basale grow into the underlying dermis and form the **hair follicle.**

    2. The deepest part of the hair follicle soon becomes club-shaped to form the **hair bulb.**

    3. The hair bulbs are invaginated by mesoderm called **hair papillae,** which are rapidly infiltrated by blood vessels and nerve endings.

    4. Epithelial cells within the hair bulb differentiate into the germinal matrix where cells proliferate, grow toward the surface, keratinize, and form the **hair shaft.** These cells also form the **internal root sheath.**

    5. Other epithelial cells of the hair follicle form the **external root sheath,** which is continuous with the epidermis.

    6. Mesodermal cells of the dermis that surround the invaginating hair follicle form the **dermal root sheath** and the **arrector pili muscle.**

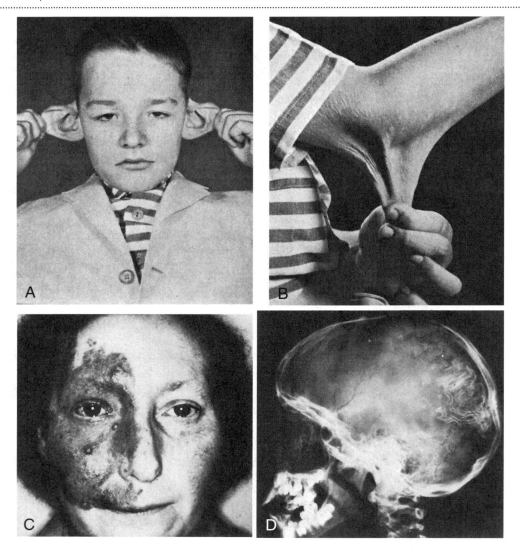

Figure 16-1.   **(A, B) Ehlers–Danlos syndrome.** Note the extremely stretchable skin of the ear and elbow region. **(C, D) Sturge-Weber syndrome.** Note the port-wine stain over the area of distribution of the trigeminal nerve (CN V). The radiograph shows calcification of the cerebral cortex closely following the cerebral convolutions (or gyri). Calcification of meningeal arteries may also be prominent. (A and B, from Smith DW, Jones KL: *Recognizable Patterns of Human Malformation*, 3rd ed. Philadelphia, WB Saunders, 1982, p 359. C and D, from Salmon HA, Lindenbaum RH: *Developmental Defects and Syndromes*. Aylesbury, England, HM & M Publishers, 1978, p 95.)

> **7.** The first fine hairs, called **lanugo hairs,** are sloughed off at birth.
>
> **8.** BMP-2 (bone morphogenetic protein), **FGF-2** (fibroblast growth factor), **sonic hedgehog,** and **Msx** (a homeobox gene) appear to be important in the development of hair.
>
> **B.** **Nails** develop from the epidermis. They first develop on the tips of the digits, then mi-

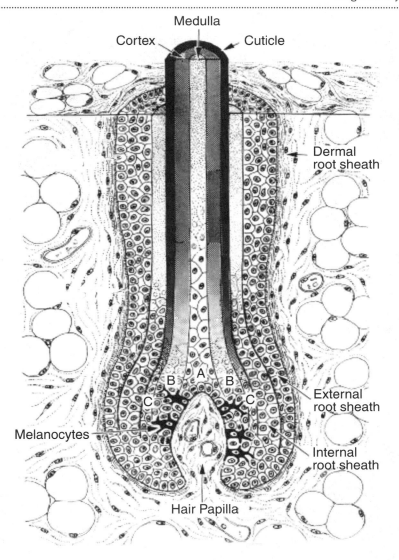

Figure 16-2.   Diagram of a hair and its follicle. The expanded lower end of the follicle contains a hair papilla. Formation and growth of the hair depend on the continuous proliferation (note the cells in mitosis) and differentiation of cells around the tip of the hair papilla. (A) Cells that give rise to the hair medulla. (B) Cells that give rise to the hair cortex. (C) Cells that give rise to the hair cuticle. Other peripheral cells give rise to the internal and external root sheath. Melanocytes contribute to hair color. (From Junqueira LC, Carneiro J, Kelley RO: *Basic Histology,* 9th ed. Stamford, CT, Appleton & Lange, 1998, p 335.)

grate to the dorsal surface, taking their innervation with them; this is why the median nerve innervates the dorsal surface of three and one-half digits (I–IV).

C. **Clinical correlations**

1. **Alopecia** is baldness resulting from an absence or faulty development of the hair follicles.

2. Hypertrichosis is an overgrowth of hair. It is frequently associated with **spina bifida occulta,** where it is seen as a patch of hair overlying the defect.

3. Pili torti is a familial disorder characterized by twisted hairs. It is seen in **Menkes' (kinky-hair) disease,** an X-linked recessive neurologic disorder.

III. MAMMARY, SWEAT, AND SEBACEOUS GLANDS. These glands are all derived from the surface ectoderm.

A. Mammary glands develop from the **mammary ridge,** a downgrowth of the epidermis (ectoderm) into the underlying dermis (mesoderm). Canalization of these epithelial downgrowths results in formation of **alveoli** and **lactiferous ducts;** the latter drain into an epithelial pit, the future **nipple.**

B. Eccrine and **apocrine sweat glands** develop from downgrowths of the epidermis into the underlying dermis.

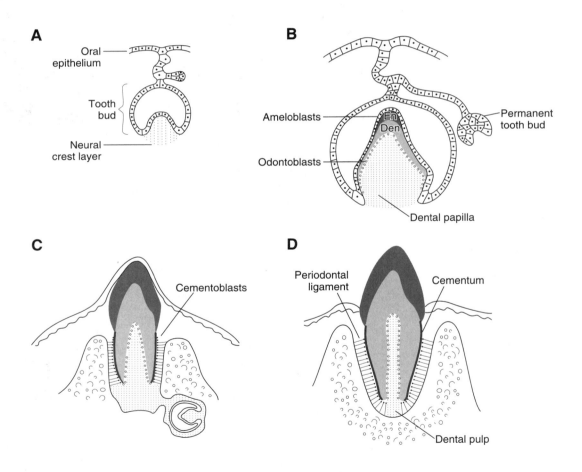

Figure 16-3. Successive stages in the development of a tooth. (A) Week 8. (B) Week 28. Note the formation of enamel (*En*) by ameloblasts and dentin (*Den*) by odontoblasts. (C) Month 6 postnatally. Note the early tooth eruption. (D) Month 18 postnatally. Note the fully erupted deciduous tooth. Ameloblasts are no longer present, which means that further enamel formation is not possible. (Modified from Dudek RW, Fix JD: *BRS Embryology,* 2nd ed. Baltimore, Williams & Wilkins, 1998, p 197.)

C. **Sebaceous glands** develop from the epithelial wall of the hair follicle and elaborate **sebum** into the hair follicles. The tarsal (meibomian) glands of the eyelids do not communicate with hair follicles.

D. Clinical correlations

1. **Gynecomastia** is a condition in which there is excessive development of the male mammary glands. It is frequently associated with Klinefelter's syndrome (47,XXY).

2. **Polymastia** is a condition in which supernumerary breasts occur along the mammary ridge.

3. **Polythelia** is a condition in which supernumerary nipples occur along the mammary ridge.

IV. **TEETH** (Figure 16-3). Teeth develop from ectoderm and an underlying layer of neural crest cells.

A. The **dental lamina** develops from the oral epithelium (ectoderm) as a downgrowth into the underlying neural crest layer. It gives rise to **tooth buds,** which develop into the **enamel organs.**

B. **Enamel organs** are derived from ectoderm. These organs develop first for the 20 deciduous teeth, then for the 32 permanent teeth. They give rise to **ameloblasts,** which produce **enamel.**

C. **Dental papilla** is formed by neural crest cells that underlie the enamel organ. It gives rise to the **odontoblasts** (which produce **predentin** and **dentin**) and **dental pulp.**

D. The **dental sac** is formed by a condensation of neural crest cells that surrounds the dental papilla. This sac gives rise to **cementoblasts** (which produce **cementum**) and the **periodontal ligaments.**

E. Clinical correlations

1. **Defective enamel formation (amelogenesis imperfecta)** is an autosomal dominant trait.

2. **Defective dentin formation (dentinogenesis imperfecta)** is an autosomal dominant trait.

3. **Discoloration of teeth** is caused by the administration of tetracycline, which stains and affects the enamel of both deciduous and permanent teeth.

17

Skeletal System

I. SKULL (Figure 17-1). The skull can be divided into two parts: the neurocranium and the viscerocranium.

A. Neurocranium. The neurocranium consists of the flat bones of the skull (cranial vault) and the base of the skull. The neurocranium develops from neural crest cells, except for the basilar part of the occipital bone, which forms from mesoderm of the occipital sclerotomes.

B. Viscerocranium. The viscerocranium consists of the bones of the face involving the pharyngeal arches, which have been discussed in Chapter 11. This part develops from neural crest cells, except for the laryngeal cartilage, which forms from mesoderm within pharyngeal arches 4 and 6.

C. Sutures

1. During fetal life and infancy, the flat bones of the skull are separated by dense connective tissue (fibrous joints) called **sutures.** There are five sutures: the **frontal suture, sagittal suture, lambdoid suture, coronal suture,** and **squamosal suture.**

2. Sutures allow the flat bones of the skull to deform during childbirth (called **molding**) and to expand during childhood as the brain grows. Molding may exert considerable tension at the "obstetric hinge" (junction of the squamous and lateral parts of the occipital bone) such that the **great cerebral vein (of Galen)** is ruptured during childbirth.

D. Fontanelles are large fibrous areas where several sutures meet. There are six fontanelles: the **anterior fontanelle, posterior fontanelle, two sphenoid fontanelles,** and **two mastoid fontanelles.**

1. The **anterior fontanelle** is the largest fontanelle and is readily palpable in the infant. It pulsates because of the underlying cerebral arteries and can be used to obtain a blood sample from the underlying **superior sagittal sinus.**

2. The **anterior fontanelle and the mastoid fontanelles** close at about **2 years of age** when the main growth of the brain ceases.

3. The **posterior fontanelle and the sphenoid fontanelles** close at approximately **6 months of age.**

E. Clinical correlations

1. **Abnormalities in the shape of the skull** may result from failure of cranial sutures to form or from premature closure of sutures (**craniosynostoses**).
   a. **Microcephaly** results from failure of the brain to grow and is usually associated with mental retardation.

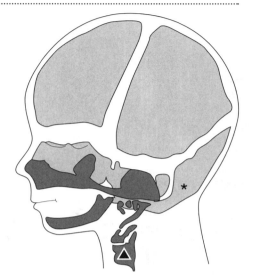

Figure 17-1. Schematic diagram of the newborn skull indicating the neurocranium (*lighter shaded area*) and the viscerocranium (*darker shaded area*). The bones of the neurocranium and viscerocranium are derived almost entirely from neural crest cells, except for the basilar part of the occipital bone (*), which forms from mesoderm of the occipital sclerotomes, and the laryngeal cartilages (▲), which form from mesoderm within pharyngeal arches 4 and 6. (Modified from Dudek RW, Fix JD: *BRS Embryology,* 2nd ed. Baltimore, Williams & Wilkins, 1998, p 201.)

> **b.** **Oxycephaly (turricephaly or acrocephaly)** is a tower-like skull caused by premature closure of the lambdoid and coronal sutures. It should be differentiated from **Crouzon's syndrome,** which is a dominant genetic condition with a presentation quite similar to that of oxycephaly but which is accompanied by malformations of the face, teeth, and ears.
>
> **c.** **Plagiocephaly** involves an asymmetric skull that is caused by premature closure of the lambdoid and coronal sutures on one side of the skull.
>
> **d.** **Scaphocephaly** is a long skull (in the anterior/posterior plane) and is caused by premature closure of the sagittal suture.

> **2.** **Temporal bone formation**
>
> **a.** **Mastoid process.** This portion of the temporal bone is absent at birth, which leaves the facial nerve (CN VII) relatively unprotected as it emerges from the stylomastoid foramen. In a difficult delivery, forceps may damage CN VII. The mastoid process forms by 2 years of age.
>
> **b.** **Petrosquamous fissure.** The petrous and squamous portions of the temporal bone are separated by the petrosquamous fissure, which opens directly into the mastoid antrum of the middle ear. This fissure, which may remain open until 20 years of age, provides a route for the spread of infection from the middle ear to the meninges.

> **3.** The **spheno-occipital joint** is a site of growth up to approximately 20 years of age.

II. VERTEBRAL COLUMN

A. **Vertebrae in general (Figure 17-2).** Mesodermal cells from the sclerotome migrate and condense around the notochord to form the **centrum,** around the neural tube to form the **vertebral arches,** and in the body wall to form the **costal processes.**

1. The centrum forms the vertebral body.

2. The vertebral arch forms the pedicles, laminae, spinous process, articular processes, and transverse processes.

3. The costal processes form the ribs.

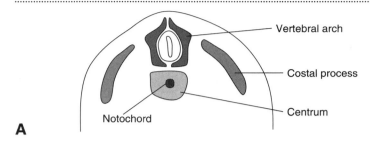

A

Vertebral arch

Costal process

Centrum

Notochord

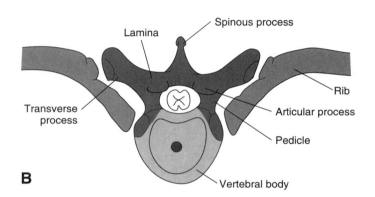

B

Lamina

Spinous process

Transverse process

Rib

Articular process

Pedicle

Vertebral body

Figure 17-2.   Schematic diagram depicting the development of a typical thoracic vertebra. (*A*) At approximately weeks 5–7, mesodermal cells from the sclerotome demonstrate three distinct condensations: a centrum, a vertebral arch, and a costal process. From 3–5 years of age, the vertebral arches fuse with each other and also fuse with the centrum. Ossification ends when the person is about 25 years of age. (*B*) In an adult, each condensation develops into distinct components of the adult vertebrae as indicated by the shading. (Modified from Dudek RW, Fix JD: *BRS Embryology*, 2nd ed. Baltimore, Williams & Wilkins, 1998, p 204.)

B. The **axis (C1)** and the **atlas (C2)** are highly modified vertebrae.

1. The **atlas** has no vertebral body.

2. The **axis** has an odontoid process (dens) that represents the vertebral body of the atlas.

C. The **sacrum** is a large triangular fusion of five sacral vertebrae that forms the posterior/superior wall of the pelvic cavity.

D. The **coccyx** is a small triangular fusion of four rudimentary vertebrae.

E. **Intersegmental position of the vertebrae (Figure 17-3)**

1. As mesodermal cells from the sclerotome migrate toward the notochord and neural tube, they split into a **cranial portion** and a **caudal portion.** The caudal portion of each sclerotome fuses with the cranial portion of the succeeding sclerotome, which results in the intersegmental position of the vertebrae. The splitting of the sclerotome is important because it allows the developing spinal nerve to have a route of access to the myotome, which it must innervate.

2. In the **cervical region,** the caudal portion of the fourth occipital sclerotome (O4) fuses with the cranial portion of the first cervical (C1) sclerotome to form the base of the occipital bone, which allows the C1 spinal nerve to exit between the base of the occipital bone and the C1 vertebrae.

F. Curves

1. The **primary curves** of the spine are the **thoracic** and **sacral curvatures** that form during the fetal period.

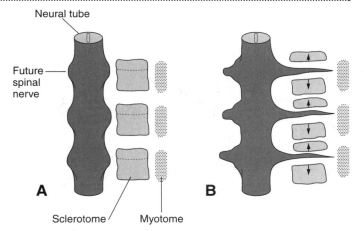

Figure 17-3. Schematic diagrams depicting the splitting of the sclerotome into caudal and cranial portions as the spinal nerves grow out to innervate the myotome. The *dotted lines* in A indicate where the sclerotome splits, thus allowing the growing spinal nerve to reach the myotome. (Modified from Dudek RW, Fix JD: *BRS Embryology,* 2nd ed. Baltimore, Williams & Wilkins, 1998, p 205.)

2. The **secondary curves** of the spine are the **cervical** and **lumbar curvatures** that form after birth as a result of lifting the head and walking, respectively.

G. Joints of the vertebral column

   1. Synovial joints
   a. The **atlanto-occipital joint** lies between C1 (atlas) and the occipital condyles.
   b. The **atlanto-axial joint** occurs between C1 (atlas) and C2 (axis).
   c. **Facets (zygapophyseal)** are joints between the inferior and superior articular facets.

   2. **Secondary cartilaginous joints (symphyses)** are the joints between the vertebral bodies in which the **intervertebral disks** play a role. An intervertebral disk consists of the **nucleus pulposus** and the **annulus fibrosus.**
   a. **Nucleus pulposus.** This is a remnant of the embryonic **notochord.** By 20 years of age, all notochordal cells have degenerated such that all notochordal vestiges in the adult are limited to just a noncellular matrix.
   b. **Annulus fibrosus.** This is an outer rim of fibrocartilage derived from mesoderm found between the vertebral bodies.

H. Clinical correlations (Figure 17-4)

   1. Congenital brevicollis (Klippel-Feil syndrome) results from fusion and shortening of the cervical vertebrae. It is associated with shortness of the neck, a low hairline, and limited motion of the head and neck.

   2. Intervertebral disk herniation involves the prolapse of the nucleus pulposus through the defective annulus fibrosus into the vertebral canal. The nucleus pulposus impinges on the spinal roots and results in root pain or radiculopathy.

   3. Spina bifida occulta results from failure of the vertebral arches to form or fuse (see Chapter 12).

   4. Spondylolisthesis occurs when the pedicles of the vertebral arches fail to fuse with the vertebral body. This allows the vertebral body to move anteriorly with respect to the vertebrae below it, causing lordosis. Congenital spondylolisthesis usually occurs at the L5–S1 vertebral level.

   5. Hemivertebrae occur when wedges of vertebrae appear that are usually situated laterally between two other vertebrae.

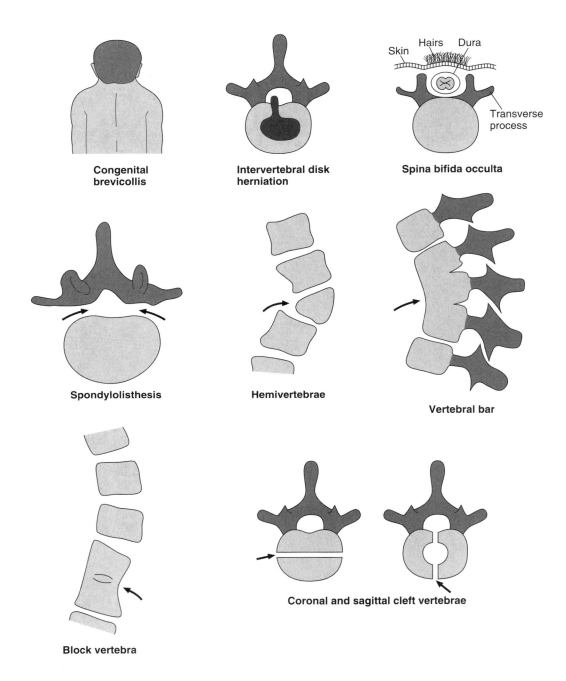

Figure 17-4. Malformations of the vertebral column. (Modified from Dudek RW, Fix JD: *BRS Embryology*, 2nd ed. Baltimore, Williams & Wilkins, 1998, p 207.)

6. **Vertebral bar** occurs when there is a localized failure of segmentation on one side of the column, usually on the posterolateral site.

7. **Block vertebra** occurs when there is a lack of separation between two or more vertebrae, usually in the lumbar region.

8. **Cleft vertebra** occurs when a fissure develops in the vertebra, usually in a coronal or sagittal plane in the lumbar region.

9. **Idiopathic scoliosis** is a lateral deviation of the vertebral column that involves both deviation and rotation of vertebral bodies.

III. RIBS

A. **Development in general.** Ribs develop from costal processes that form at all vertebral levels. However, only in the thoracic region do the costal processes grow into ribs.

B. Clinical correlations

1. **Accessory lumbar ribs** are the most common rib anomalies.

2. **Accessory cervical ribs.** These ribs are attached to the C7 vertebra and may either end freely or be attached to the thoracic cage. Accessory cervical ribs may exert pressure on the lower trunk of the brachial plexus and subclavian artery, causing **superior thoracic outlet syndrome.**

IV. STERNUM

A. **Development in general.** The sternum develops from two sternal bars that form in the ventral body wall independent of the ribs and clavicle. The sternal bars fuse with each other in a craniocaudal direction to form the **manubrium, body,** and **xiphoid process** by week 8.

B. Clinical correlations

1. **Sternal cleft** occurs when the sternal bars do not fuse completely. It is fairly common and, if small, is generally of no clinical significance.

2. **Pectus excavatum (funnel chest)** is the most common chest anomaly; it consists of a depression in the chest wall, which may extend from the manubrium to the xiphoid process. Early surgical intervention is generally recommended for patients with this anomaly, not only to improve cosmetic appearance (drooped shoulders, a protuberant abdomen), but also to alleviate cardiopulmonary restriction and scoliosis.

V. BONES OF THE LIMBS AND LIMB GIRDLES

A. Development in general (see Chapters 19 and 20)

1. The bones of the limb and limb girdles develop from condensations of lateral plate mesoderm within the limb buds. The limb buds are visible at week 4 of development; the upper limb appears first. The limbs are well differentiated at week 8.

2. The limb tip contains the **apical ectodermal ridge,** which exerts an inductive influence on limb growth and development.

B. Clinical correlations

1. **Amelia,** an absence of one or two extremities, may result from the use of the teratogen **thalidomide.**

2. **Polydactyly** is an autosomal dominant disorder that is characterized by the presence of extra digits on the hands and feet.

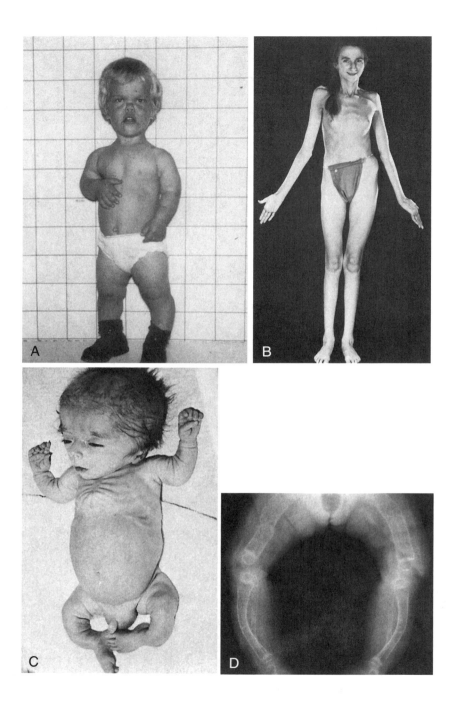

Figure 17-5. (A) Boy with achondroplasia. Note the short stature, short limbs and fingers, normal length of the trunk, bowed legs, relatively large head, prominent forehead, and deep nasal bridge. (B) Girl with Marfan's syndrome. Note the unusually tall stature, exceptionally long limbs, and arachnodactyly (elongated hands and feet with very slender digits). (C) Infant with osteogenesis imperfecta. Note the short, bowed lower limbs. (D) Radiograph of the lower limbs in a patient with osteogenesis imperfecta. Note the multiple fractures that result in an accordion-like shortening of the limb. (A, from Moore KL, Persaud TVN: The *Developing Human: Clinically Oriented Embryology*, 6th ed. Philadelphia, WB Saunders, 1998, p 179. B, C, and D, from Salmon MA, Lindenbaum RH: *Developmental Defects and Syndromes*. Aylesbury, England, HM & M Publishers, 1978, pp 172 and 251.)

3. Syndactyly (webbed fingers or toes), the most common limb anomaly, results from failure of the hand or foot webs to degenerate between the digits.

4. Holt-Oram syndrome (heart-hand syndrome), an autosomal dominant condition associated with chromosome 12, causes anomalies of the upper limb and heart.

VI. OSTEOGENESIS. Osteogenesis occurs through the conversion of pre-existing connective tissue (mesoderm) into bone, a process called **ossification.** During development, two types of ossification occur:

A. **Intramembranous ossification** occurs in the embryo when mesoderm condenses into sheets of highly vascular connective tissue, which then **directly** forms a primary ossification center. **Bones that form via intramembranous ossification** are the frontal bone, parietal bones, intraparietal part of the occipital bone, maxilla, zygomatic bone, squamous part of the temporal bone, palatine, vomer, and mandible.

B. **Endochondral ossification** occurs in the embryo when mesoderm first forms a hyaline cartilage model, which subsequently develops a primary ossification center at the diaphysis. **Bones that form via endochondral ossification** are the ethmoid bone, sphenoid bone, petrous and mastoid parts of the temporal bone, basilar part of the occipital bone, incus, malleus, stapes, styloid process, hyoid bone, bones of the limbs, limb girdles, vertebrae, sternum, and ribs.

VII. GENERAL SKELETAL ABNORMALITIES

A. **Achondroplasia (Figure 17-5A)** is the most prevalent form of dwarfism.

1. Achondroplasia is caused by a mutation in the gene for the **FGF-3 receptor** (fibroblast growth factor) on chromosome 4p.

2. Pathologic changes are observed at the **epiphyseal growth plate,** where the zones of proliferation and hypertrophy are narrow and disorganized. Horizontal struts of bone eventually grow into the growth plate and "seal" the bone, thus preventing bone growth.

3. Mental function is not affected.

4. Chances of achondroplasia increase with increasing paternal age.

B. **Marfan's syndrome (Figure 17-5B)** is a genetic defect that involves the protein **fibrillin,** an essential component of **elastic fibers.** People with Marfan's syndrome are unusually tall with exceptionally long limbs; they also have ectopia lentis (dislocation of the lens).

C. **Osteogenesis imperfecta (see Figure 17-5 C, D)** is caused by a **deficiency in type I collagen.** It is characterized by extreme bone fragility; spontaneous fractures occur when the fetus is still in the womb. Blue sclera of the eye is another characteristic of this disorder. Severe forms of osteogenesis imperfecta are fatal in utero or during the early neonatal period. Milder forms may be confused with child abuse.

D. **Acromegaly** results from **hyperpituitarism.** It is characterized by a large jaw, large hands and feet, and sometimes by gigantism.

E. **Cretinism** (see Chapter 11) occurs when there is a deficiency in **fetal thyroid hormone (T3 and T4) or thyroid agenesis.** It results in growth retardation, skeletal abnormalities, mental retardation, and neurologic disorders. Cretinism is rare except in areas where there is a lack of **iodine** in the water and soil.

18

Muscular System

I. SKELETAL MUSCLE

A. Molecular events

    1. **Mesodermal (mesenchymal) cells** within somites become committed to a muscle-forming cell line (through a poorly understood mechanism) to form **myogenic cells.**

    2. Stimulated by fibroblast growth factor **(FGF)** and transforming growth factor **(TGF-β)**, myogenic cells enter the cell cycle (i.e., undergo mitosis).

    3. Myogenic cells begin to express **MyoD** (a helix–loop–helix transcription factor), which removes the myogenic cells from the cell cycle (i.e., mitosis stops) and switches on **muscle-specific genes** to form postmitotic **myoblasts.**

    4. Myoblasts begin to synthesize **actin** and **myosin;** in addition, myoblasts fuse with each other to form multinucleated **myotubes.**

    5. Myotubes synthesize **actin, myosin, troponin, tropomyosin,** and **other muscle proteins;** these proteins aggregate into **myofibrils,** at which stage the cells are called **muscle fibers.**

    6. Because muscle fibers are postmitotic, further growth is accomplished by means of **satellite cells,** through a poorly understood mechanism.

B. **Paraxial mesoderm** is a thick plate of mesoderm on each side of the midline. This thick plate becomes organized into segments known as **somitomeres,** which form in a craniocaudal sequence.

    1. **Somitomeres 1–7** do not form somites but contribute mesoderm to the head and neck region (**pharyngeal arches**).

    2. The **remaining somitomeres** further condense in a craniocaudal sequence to form 42–44 pairs of somites of the trunk region. The somites closest to the caudal end eventually disappear to give a final count of approximately **35 pairs of somites.**

    3. Somites further differentiate into the **sclerotome** (cartilage and bone component), **myotome** (muscle component), and **dermatome** (dermis of skin component).

C. **Head and neck musculature** (see Chapter 11) is derived from somitomeres 1–7 of the head and neck region, which participate in the formation of the pharyngeal arches.

    1. **Extraocular muscles** are derived from somitomeres 1, 2, 3, and 5.

        a. Somitomeres 1, 2, and 3 are called **preotic myotomes.**

        b. Extraocular muscles are innervated by cranial nerve (CN) III, CN IV, and CN VI.

2. Tongue muscles are derived from **occipital myotomes** innervated by CN XII.

D. Trunk musculature (Figure 18-1) is derived from myotomes in the trunk region. Each myotome partitions into a dorsal **epimere** and a ventral **hypomere.**

    1. Epimeres develop into the intrinsic back muscles (e.g., erector spinae). They are innervated by the dorsal ramus of a spinal nerve.

    2. Hypomeres develop into the prevertebral, intercostal, and abdominal muscles. They are innervated by the ventral ramus of a spinal nerve.

E. Limb musculature (see Figure 18-1) is derived from myotomes (somites) in the upper and lower limb bud regions. This mesoderm migrates into the limb bud and forms a **posterior condensation** and an **anterior condensation.**

    1. The posterior condensation develops into the **extensor and supinator musculature of the upper limb** and the **extensor and abductor musculature of the lower limb.**

    2. The anterior condensation develops into the **flexor and pronator musculature of the upper limb** and the **flexor and adductor musculature of the lower limb.**

II. SMOOTH MUSCLE of the gastrointestinal tract and the tunica media of blood vessels is derived from mesoderm.

III. CARDIAC MUSCLE is derived from mesoderm that surrounds the primitive heart tube and becomes the myocardium.

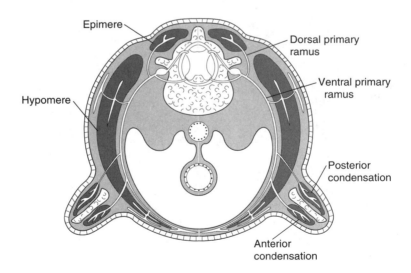

Figure 18-1.   Drawing of a transverse section through the thorax and limb bud, showing the muscles of the epimere, hypomere, and limb bud. The limb bud musculature develops from mesoderm of various myotomes. The epimeric muscles are innervated by dorsal primary rami, and the hypomeric and limb muscles are innervated by ventral primary rami of spinal nerves. (From Dudek RW, Fix JD: *BRS Embryology*, 2nd ed. Baltimore, Williams & Wilkins, 1998, p 214.)

IV. CLINICAL CORRELATIONS

A. **Prune belly syndrome** occurs when the **abdominal musculature** is absent or very hypoplastic, most likely involving cells of the hypomere.

B. **Poland's syndrome** is a relatively uncommon chest anomaly that is characterized by the **partial or complete absence of the pectoralis major muscle.** Affected individuals may demonstrate partial agenesis of the ribs and sternum, mammary gland aplasia, or absence of the latissimus dorsi and serratus anterior muscles.

C. **Congenital torticollis (wryneck)** occurs when the **sternocleidomastoid muscle is abnormally shortened** causing rotation and tilting of the head. It may be caused by injury to the sternocleidomastoid muscle during childbirth, formation of a hematoma, and eventual fibrosis of the muscle.

D. **Duchenne muscular dystrophy (DMD)**

  1. The characteristic dysfunction in DMD is **progressive muscle weakness and wasting.** Death occurs as a result of cardiac or respiratory failure, usually in a person's late teens or 20s.

  2. DMD is caused by a **genetic mutation.**

   a. The DMD gene, located on the **short (p) arm of chromosome X in band 21 (Xp21),** encodes for a protein called **dystrophin.** This protein anchors the cytoskeleton (actin) of skeletal muscle cells to the extracellular matrix through a transmembrane protein (α-dystroglycan and β-dystroglycan) and stabilizes the cell membrane.

   b. A mutation of the DMD gene destroys the ability of dystrophin to anchor actin to the extracellular matrix.

  3. DMD demonstrates an **X-linked recessive inheritance,** that is, males who have only one defective copy of the DMD gene from the mother have the disease.

19
Upper Limb

I. OVERVIEW OF DEVELOPMENT

A. **Lateral plate mesoderm** migrates into the limb bud and condenses along the central axis to eventually form the **vasculature** and the **skeletal components** of the upper limb.

B. **Mesoderm from the somites** migrates into the limb bud and condenses to eventually form the **musculature** of the upper limb.

C. Apical ectodermal ridge (AER)

   1. The AER is a ridge of thickened ectoderm at the apex of the limb bud.

   2. The AER produces **fibroblast growth factor (FGF),** which interacts with the underlying mesoderm to promote outgrowth of the limb by stimulating mitosis and preventing terminal differentiation of the underlying mesoderm.

   3. This ridge expresses the **Wnt7 gene** that directs the organization of the limb bud along the dorsal–ventral axis.

D. Zone of polarizing activity (ZPA)

   1. The ZPA consists of mesodermal cells located at the base of the limb bud.

   2. This zone produces **sonic hedgehog** (a diffusible protein encoded by a segment polarity gene), which directs the organization of the limb bud along the anterior–posterior polar axis and patterning of the digits.

   3. Sonic hedgehog activates the gene **for bone morphogenetic protein (BMP)** and the **Hoxd-9, Hoxd-10, Hoxd-11, Hoxd-12, and Hoxd-13 genes.**

   4. **Retinoic acid** also plays a significant role in limb polarization.

E. **Digit formation** occurs as a result of selected **apoptosis (cell death)** within the AER such that five separate regions of AER remain at the tips of the future digits. The exact mechanism is poorly understood, although **BMP, Msx-1, and the retinoic acid receptor** may play a role.

II. VASCULATURE

A. **Aortic arch 4** forms the proximal part of the right subclavian artery.

B. The **7th intersegmental artery** forms the distal part of the right subclavian artery and the entire left subclavian artery.

C. The **subclavian artery (right and left)** continues into the limb bud as the **axis artery,** which ends in a **terminal plexus** near the tip of the limb bud.

Week 5

Week 6

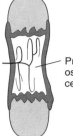

Primary
ossification
center

Weeks 7–9

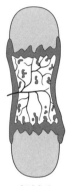

At birth

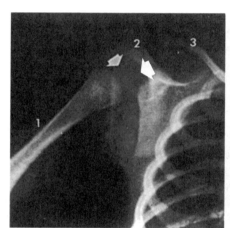

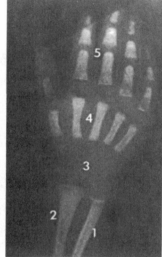

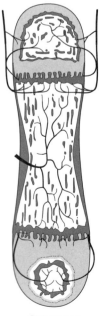

Childhood

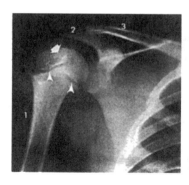

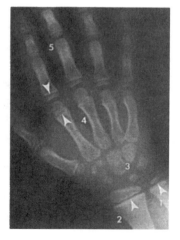

D. The **terminal plexus** participates in the formation of the **deep palmar arch** and the **superficial palmar arch.**

E. Axis artery

  1. This artery initially sprouts the **posterior interosseous artery** and the **median artery** (which is reduced to an unnamed vessel in the adult).

  2. The axis artery later sprouts the **radial artery** and the **ulnar artery.**

  3. The artery persists in the adult as the axillary artery, brachial artery, anterior interosseous artery, and deep palmar arch.

III. SKELETAL COMPONENTS (Figure 19-1)

A. **Lateral plate mesoderm** forms the **scapula, clavicle, humerus, radius, ulnar, carpals, metacarpals,** and **phalanges.**

B. **Ossification.** All the bones of the upper limb undergo endochondral ossification; however, the clavicle undergoes both membranous and endochondral ossification.

C. Timing of bone formation

  1. **Week 5:** Lateral plate mesoderm within the limb bud condenses.

  2. **Week 6:** Condensed mesoderm chondrifies to form a hyaline cartilage model of the upper limb bones.

  3. **Week 7:** Primary ossification centers are seen in the clavicle, humerus, radius, and ulnar bones. The clavicle is the first bone in the entire body to ossify.

  4. **Week 9 to birth:** Primary ossification centers are seen in the scapula, metacarpals, and phalanges.

  5. **Childhood:** Secondary ossification centers form in the epiphyseal ends. All carpal bones begin ossification.

Figure 19-1.   Bone formation in the upper limb.

    Week 5. Lateral plate mesoderm condenses (*hatched*). **Week 6.** Hyaline cartilage (*light shading*) model of future bones forms. **Weeks 7–9.** Primary ossification centers within the diaphysis appear such that bone (*dark shading*) forms (osteogenesis).

    At birth. The diaphysis consists of bone (*dark shading*), whereas the epiphysis remains hyaline cartilage (*light shading*). This is important to note when interpreting radiographs of newborns. The radiograph of a newborn at the shoulder region (*1* = humerus; *2* = acromion; *3* = clavicle) shows the portion of the hyaline cartilage model that has been replaced by radiodense bone (white). Note that the epiphyseal end of the humerus (*white arrow*) is still hyaline cartilage at birth and, therefore, will appear radiolucent (dark). The radiograph of a newborn arm and hand shows the portion of the hyaline cartilage model that has been replaced by radiodense bone (white) in the ulnar (*1*), radius (*2*), metacarpals (*4*), and phalanges (*5*). Note the epiphyseal ends of these bones (*1, 2, 4, 5*). All of the carpal bones (*3*) are still hyaline cartilage and, therefore, are radiolucent (dark). The carpal bones of the wrist begin to ossify much later in childhood.

    Childhood. During childhood, secondary ossification centers form in the epiphyseal ends of the bones. During childhood and adolescence, the growth in length of long bones occurs at the epiphyseal growth plate. Note the radiograph of a 6-year-old child at the shoulder region. *1* = humerus; *2* = acromion; *3* = clavicle. Because secondary ossification centers are present within the epiphyseal ends of the humerus, the head of the humerus is now radiodense (*white arrow*) and the epiphyseal growth plate (*arrowheads*) where hyaline cartilage is present remains radiolucent (dark). This should not be confused with a bone fracture. The radiograph showing the wrist and hand of a 6-year-old child demonstrates the radiodense bone (white) within the diaphyseal and epiphyseal portions of the ulnar bone (*1*) and radius bone (*2*) as well as the radiolucent (dark) epiphyseal growth plates (*arrowheads*), which are hyaline cartilage. The diaphyseal and epiphyseal portions of the metacarpals (*4*) and phalanges (*5*), as well as their epiphyseal growth plates (*arrowheads*), can also be observed. Note that the carpal bones (*3*) have begun to ossify. (From Dudek RW, Fix JD: *BRS Embryology,* 2nd ed. Baltimore, Williams & Wilkins, 1998, p 220.)

20
Lower Limb

I. OVERVIEW OF DEVELOPMENT

A. **Lateral plate mesoderm** migrates into the limb bud and condenses along the central axis to eventually form the **vasculature** and the **skeletal components** of the upper limb.

B. **Mesoderm from the somites** migrates into the limb bud and condenses to eventually form the **musculature** of the upper limb.

C. Apical ectodermal ridge (AER)

    1. The AER is a ridge of thickened ectoderm at the apex of the limb bud.

    2. The AER produces **fibroblast growth factor (FGF),** which interacts with the underlying mesoderm to promote outgrowth of the limb by stimulating mitosis and preventing terminal differentiation of the underlying mesoderm.

    3. The AER expresses the **Wnt7 gene,** which directs the organization of the limb bud along the dorsal/ventral axis.

D. Zone of polarizing activity (ZPA)

    1. The ZPA consists of mesodermal cells located at the base of the limb bud.

    2. This zone produces **sonic hedgehog** (a diffusible protein encoded by a segment polarity gene), which directs the organization of the limb bud along the anterior–posterior polar axis and patterning of the digits.

    3. Sonic hedgehog activates the gene for **bone morphogenetic protein (BMP)** and the **Hoxd-9, Hoxd-10, Hoxd-11, Hoxd-12, and Hoxd-13 genes.**

    4. **Retinoic acid** also plays a significant role in limb polarization.

E. **Digit formation** occurs as a result of selected **apoptosis (cell death)** within the AER in such a way that five separate regions of AER remain at the tips of the future digits. The exact mechanism is poorly understood, although **BMP, Msx-1, and retinoic acid receptor** may play a role.

II. VASCULATURE

A. The **umbilical artery** gives rise to the **axis artery** of the lower limb, which ends in a **terminal plexus** near the tip of the limb bud.

B. The **terminal plexus** participates in the formation of the **deep plantar arch.**

C. Axis artery

    1. This artery sprouts the **anterior tibial artery** (which continues as the **dorsalis pedis**

artery) and the **posterior tibial artery** (which terminates as the **medial plantar artery** and **lateral plantar artery**).

2. Although most of the axis artery regresses, it ultimately persists in the adult as the **inferior gluteal artery, sciatic artery** (accompanying the sciatic nerve), proximal part of the **popliteal artery,** and distal part of the **peroneal artery.**

D. External iliac artery

1. This artery gives rise to the **femoral artery** of the lower limb, which constitutes a separate second arterial channel into the lower limb, which connects to the axis artery.

2. The femoral artery sprouts the **profunda femoris artery.**

III. SKELETAL COMPONENTS (Figure 20-1)

A. Lateral plate mesoderm forms the **ilium, ischium, pubis, femur, tibia, fibula, tarsals, metatarsals,** and **phalanges.**

B. Ossification. All bones of the lower limb undergo endochondral ossification.

C. Timing of bone formation

1. **Week 5:** Lateral plate mesoderm condenses within the limb bud.

2. **Week 6:** Condensed mesoderm chondrifies to form a hyaline cartilage model of all the lower limb bones.

3. **Week 7:** Primary ossification centers are seen in the femur and tibia.

4. **Week 9 to birth:** Primary ossification centers are seen in the ilium, ischium, pubis, fibula, calcaneus, talus, metatarsals, and phalanges. The ossification of the calcaneus (weeks 16–20) is used medicolegally to establish maturity.

5. **Childhood:** Secondary ossification centers form in the epiphyseal ends. The remaining tarsal bones begin ossification.

IV. MUSCULATURE

A. The lower limb bud site lies opposite somites L1, L2, L3, L4, L5, S1, and S2. During week 5, mesoderm from these somites (myotomes) migrates into the limb bud and forms a **posterior condensation** and an **anterior condensation.**

B. The mesoderm of these condensations differentiates into myoblasts. The condensations then split into anatomically recognizable muscles of the lower limb; little is known about this process.

1. The **posterior condensation,** in general, gives rise to the **extensor and abductor musculature.**

2. The **anterior condensation,** in general, gives rise to the **flexor and adductor musculature.**

V. NERVES (LUMBOSACRAL PLEXUS)

A. Local cell biologic messages produced at the base of the limb bud guide the early nerve fibers into the limb bud; the muscle themselves do not provide any specific target messages to the ingrowing nerve fibers.

B. Ventral primary rami from L2, L3, L4, L5, S1, S2, and S3 arrive at the base of the limb bud and divide into **posterior divisions** and **anterior divisions.**

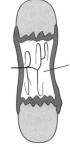

Week 5　　**Week 6**

Primary
ossification
center

Weeks 7–9

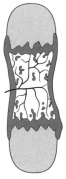

At birth

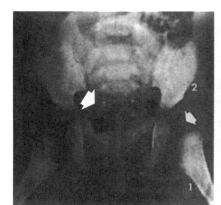

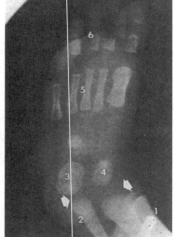

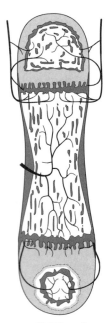

Childhood

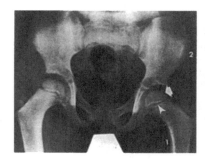

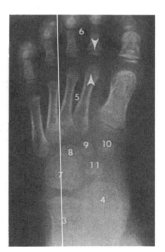

1. Posterior divisions
   a. These divisions grow into the posterior condensation of mesoderm.
   b. Posterior divisions will form the **superior gluteal nerve (L4, L5, S1), inferior gluteal nerve (L5, S1, S2), femoral nerve (L2, L3, L4)**, and **common peroneal nerve (L4, L5, S1, S2),** thus innervating all the muscles that form from the posterior condensation.

2. Anterior divisions
   a. Anterior divisions grow into the anterior condensation of mesoderm.
   b. These divisions will form the **tibial nerve (L4, L5, S1, S2, S3)** and the **obturator nerve (L2, L3, L4),** thus innervating all the muscles that form from the anterior condensation.

VI. ROTATION

A. The lower limb buds appear in **week 4** (about 4 days after the upper limb bud) as small bulges oriented in a **coronal plane.**

B. The lower limb buds undergo a horizontal flexion in **week 6** so that they are now oriented in a **parasagittal plane.**

C. The lower limbs **rotate medially 90°** during weeks 6–8 so that the knee points anteriorly, the extensor compartment lies anteriorly, and the flexor compartment lies posteriorly. This rotation causes the originally straight segmental pattern of innervation (dermatomes) to be modified slightly in the adult **(Figure 20-2).**

D. Note that the **upper limbs rotate laterally 90°,** whereas the **lower limbs rotate medially 90°.** This rotation sets up the following anatomic situations:

1. The flexor compartment of the upper limb is anterior, whereas the flexor compartment of the lower limb is posterior.

Figure 20-1.   Bone formation in the lower limb.

Week 5. Lateral plate mesoderm condenses (*hatched*). **Week 6.** Hyaline cartilage (*light shading*) model of future bones forms. **Weeks 7–9.** Primary ossification centers within the diaphysis appear such that bone (*dark shading*) forms (osteogenesis).

At birth. The diaphysis consists of bone (*dark shading*), whereas the epiphysis remains hyaline cartilage. This is important to note when interpreting radiographs of newborns. The radiograph of a newborn at the hip region (*1* = femur; *2* = ilium) shows the portions of the hyaline cartilage model that have been replaced by radiodense bone (white). Note that the epiphyseal end of the femur (*white arrow*) is still hyaline cartilage at birth and will therefore appear radiolucent (dark). The radiograph of a newborn at the ankle and foot shows the portions of the hyaline cartilage model that have been replaced by radiodense bone (white) in the tibia (*1*), fibula (*2*), calcaneus (*3*), talus (*4*), metatarsals (*5*), and phalanges (*6*). Note that the epiphyseal ends of the tibia and fibula are still cartilage and are, therefore, radiolucent (*white arrows*).

Childhood. During childhood, secondary ossification centers form in the epiphyseal ends of the bones. During childhood and adolescence, the growth in length of long bones occurs at the epiphyseal growth plate. Note the radiograph of a 6-year-old child at the hip region (*1* = femur; *2* = ilium). Because secondary ossification centers are present within the epiphyseal ends, the head of the femur is now radiodense (*white arrow*), and the epiphyseal growth plate (*arrowhead*) where hyaline cartilage is present remains radiolucent (dark). This should not be confused with a bone fracture. On the radiograph of a 6-year-old child at the foot, the diaphyseal and epiphyseal portions of the metatarsals (*5*) and phalanges (*6*) as well as their epiphyseal growth plates (*arrowheads*) can be observed. The remaining tarsal bones have begun to ossify. *3* = calcaneus; *4* = talus; *7* = cuboid; *8* = lateral cuneiform; *9* = intermediate cuneiform; *10* = medial cuneiform; *11* = navicular. (From Dudek RW, Fix JD: *BRS Embryology*, 2nd ed. Baltimore, Williams & Wilkins, 1998, p 230.)

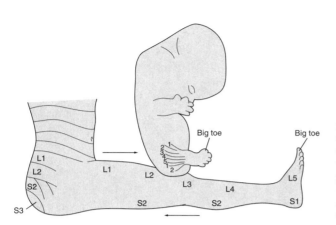

Figure 20-2. Dermatome pattern in the adult lower limb and limb bud. The 90° medial rotation of the lower limb bud causes the originally straight segmental pattern of innervation in the embryo to be somewhat modified (i.e., "twisted in a spiral") such that the dermatome pattern in the adult is altered. However, an orderly dermatome pattern can still be recognized in the adult if the lower limb is positioned in a parasagittal plane with the big toe pointing superiorly (as shown). The dermatomes from L1 can be counted distally down the superior border of the lower limb (*arrow*) to L5 and then back proximally up the inferior border of the lower limb (*arrow*) to S2. (From Dudek RW, Fix JD: *BRS Embryology,* 2nd ed. Baltimore, Williams & Wilkins, 1998, p 234.)

2. The extensor compartment of the upper limb is posterior, whereas the extensor compartment of the lower limb is anterior.

3. Flexion at the wrist joint is analogous to plantar flexion at the ankle joint.

4. Extension at the wrist joint is analogous to dorsiflexion at the ankle joint.

21

Pregnancy

I. ENDOCRINOLOGY OF PREGNANCY

A. Human chorionic gonadotropin (HCG)

1. Definition. HCG is a glycoprotein hormone produced by the **syncytiotrophoblast.** It stimulates the production of progesterone by the corpus luteum (i.e., it maintains the function of the corpus luteum). HCG is detectable throughout a pregnancy.

2. Pregnancy tests. HCG can be assayed in **maternal blood at day 8 or in maternal urine at day 10** using a radioimmunoassay with antibodies directed against the β-subunit of HCG. The presence of HCG in maternal urine is the basis of the early pregnancy test kits purchased over the counter.

3. Quantitative HCG dating of pregnancy. During weeks 1–6 of a normal pregnancy, HCG levels increase by about 70% every 48 hours:

0–2 weeks:	0–250 mIU/ml
2–4 weeks:	100–5000 mIU/ml
1–2 months:	4000–200,000 mIU/ml
2–3 months:	8000–100,000 mIU/ml
2nd trimester:	4000–75,000 mIU/ml
3rd trimester:	1000–5000 mIU/ml

4. Other tests using HCG levels. Low HCG levels may predict a spontaneous abortion or indicate an ectopic pregnancy. Elevated HCG levels may indicate a multiple pregnancy, hydatidiform mole, or gestational trophoblastic neoplasia.

B. Human placental lactogen (HPL)

1. HPL, a protein hormone produced by the **placenta,** induces lipolysis, thus elevating free fatty acid levels in the mother. It is considered to be the "growth hormone" of the latter half of pregnancy.

2. HPL can be assayed in **maternal blood at week 6.**

3. HPL levels vary with placental mass (i.e., higher than normal levels may indicate a multiple pregnancy) and rapidly disappear from maternal blood after delivery.

C. Prolactin (PRL)

1. PRL is a protein hormone produced by the **maternal adenohypophysis, fetal adenohypophysis,** and **decidual tissue of the uterus.** It prepares the mammary glands for lactation.

    2. PRL can be assayed in **maternal blood throughout pregnancy** or in **amniotic fluid in late pregnancy.** Near term, PRL levels rise to a maximum of about 100 ng/ml (normal nonpregnant PRL levels range between 8 and 25 ng/ml).

D. **Progesterone** is a steroid hormone produced by the **corpus luteum** until week 8 and then by the **placenta** until birth.

    1. Progesterone prepares the **endometrium** for implantation (nidation) and maintains the endometrium.

    2. It is used by the fetal adrenal cortex as a **precursor for corticosteroid synthesis.**

    3. It is used by the fetal testes as a **precursor for testosterone synthesis.**

E. Estrone, estradiol, and estriol

    1. These steroid hormones are produced by a complex series of steps involving the **maternal liver, placenta, fetal adrenal gland,** and **fetal liver.**
        a. Cholesterol from the maternal liver is converted to pregnenolone by the placenta.
        b. Pregnenolone is converted to pregnenolone sulfate.
        c. Pregnenolone sulfate is converted to dehydroepiandrosterone sulfate (DHEA-SO_4) by the fetal adrenal gland.
        d. DHEA-SO_4 is converted to estrone and estradiol by the placenta.
        e. DHEA-SO_4 is also converted to 16-α-hydroxy DHEA-SO_4 by the fetal liver.
        f. 16-α-hydroxy DHEA-SO_4 is converted to estriol by the placenta.

    2. **Estrone** is a fairly weak estrogen.

    3. **Estradiol** is the most potent estrogen.

    4. **Estriol** is a very weak estrogen but is produced in very high amounts during pregnancy.
        a. Estriol can be assayed in **maternal blood** (it shows a distinct diurnal variation with peak amounts early in the morning) and in **maternal urine** (24-hour urine sample shows no diurnal variation). Significant amounts of estriol are produced in the third month (i.e., early second trimester) and continue to rise until birth.
        b. Maternal urinary levels of estriol have long been recognized as a **reliable index of fetal–placental function** because estriol production depends on a normal functioning fetal adrenal cortex, fetal liver, and placenta.

II. **PREGNANCY DATING.** The **estimated date of confinement (EDC)** is based on the assumption that a woman has a 28-day cycle with ovulation on day 14 or day 15. In general, the duration of a normal pregnancy is **280 days (40 weeks) from the first day of the last menstrual period (LMP).** A common method to determine the EDC (Nägele's rule) is to count back 3 months from the first day of the LMP and then add 1 year and 7 days; this method is reasonably accurate in women with regular menstrual cycles.

III. **PREGNANCY MILESTONES**

A. The **first trimester** extends from the last menstrual period through week 12. Important events are as follows:

    1. At days 8–10, a positive result on a pregnancy test is obtained by HCG assay.

    2. At week 12, the uterine fundus is palpable at the pubic symphysis, and Doppler fetal heart rate is first audible.

B. The **second trimester** extends from the end of the first trimester through week 27. Important events are as follows:

1. At weeks 14–18, **amniocentesis** is performed when there is a risk of fetal chromosomal abnormalities.

2. At week 16, the uterine fundus is palpable midway between the pubic symphysis and the umbilicus.

3. At weeks 16–18, first fetal movements occur (**quickening**) in a woman who has had one or more previous pregnancies.

4. At weeks 17–20, fetal heart rate is audible with a fetoscope.

5. At week 18, female and male external genitalia can be distinguished by ultrasound (i.e., **sex determination**).

6. At weeks 18–20, the first fetal movements occur (**quickening**) in a woman's first pregnancy.

7. At week 20, the uterine fundus is palpable at the umbilicus.

8. At weeks 25–27, the lungs become capable of respiration; **surfactant** is produced by type II pneumocytes. There is a 70%–80% chance of survival in infants born at the end of the second trimester. If death occurs, it is generally as a result of lung immaturity and resultant respiratory distress syndrome (hyaline membrane disease).

9. At week 27, the fetus weighs approximately 1000 g (a little more than 2 lb).

C. The **third trimester** extends from the end of the second trimester until term or week 40. Important events are as follows:

1. Pupillary light reflex is present.

2. Descent of the fetal head to the pelvic inlet (called **lightening**) occurs.

3. Rupture of the amniochorionic membrane occurs, with labor usually beginning about 24 hours later.

4. The fetus weighs about 3300 g (about 7–7.5 lb).

IV. PRENATAL DIAGNOSTIC PROCEDURES are indicated in approximately 8% of all pregnancies.

A. **Ultrasonography** is commonly used to date pregnancy, to diagnose a multiple pregnancy, to assess fetal growth, to determine placenta location, to determine the position and lie of the fetus, to detect certain congenital anomalies, and to monitor needle or catheter insertion during amniocentesis and chorionic villus biopsy.

1. In obstetric ultrasonography, 2.25–5.0 mHz frequencies are used for good tissue differentiation.

2. The term **anechoic** refers to tissues with few or no echoes (e.g., bladder, brain, cavities, amniotic fluid); the term **echogenic** refers to tissues with a high capacity to reflect ultrasound.

3. **B–scan ultrasonography** consists of an **A-mode** and an **M-mode** (which provide precise measurements) and a **time position scan** with a permanent record of cinephotography.

4. **Real-time ultrasonography** provides an easy, immediate, and definitive demonstration of fetal life.

B. **Amniocentesis is a transabdominal sampling of amniotic fluid and fetal cells.** It is performed at weeks 14–18 for the following indications: the woman is over 35 years of age, a previous child has a chromosomal anomaly, one parent is a known carrier of a translocation or inversion, one or both parents are known carriers of an X-linked recessive or autosomal recessive trait, or there is a history of a neuron tube defect. The sample obtained is used in the following studies:

1. **α-Fetoprotein assay,** used to diagnose neural tube defects

2. **Spectrophotometric assay of bilirubin,** used to diagnose hemolytic disease of the newborn (i.e., erythroblastosis fetalis) due to Rh-incompatibility

3. **Lecithin-sphingomyelin (L/S) ratio and phosphatidylglycerol assay,** used to determine the lung maturity of the fetus

4. **DNA analysis.** Numerous DNA methodologies are available [e.g., karyotype analysis, Southern blotting, or restriction fragment length polymorphism (RFLP) analysis] to diagnose chromosomal abnormalities and single gene defects.

C. **Chorionic villus biopsy** is a transabdominal or transcervical sampling of the chorionic villi to obtain a large amount of **fetal cells** for DNA analysis. It is performed at weeks 6–11 (i.e., much earlier than amniocentesis).

D. **Percutaneous umbilical blood sampling (PUBS)** is a sampling of **fetal blood** from the umbilical cord.

V. FETAL DISTRESS DURING LABOR (INTRAPARTUM FETAL DISTRESS) is defined in terms of **fetal hypoxia** and measured by changes in either **fetal heart rate (FHR)** or **fetal scalp capillary pH.**

A. The normal baseline FHR is 120–160 beats/min; fetal hypoxia causes a decrease in FHR (or **fetal bradycardia**), that is, a FHR of less than 120 beats/min.

B. Normal fetal scalp capillary pH is 7.25–7.35; fetal hypoxia causes a decrease in pH, that is, a pH of less than 7.20.

VI. APGAR SCORE

A. The APGAR score assesses five characteristics in the newborn—appearance, pulse, grimace, activity, and respiratory effort—in order to determine which infants need resuscitation.

B. It is performed at 1 minute and 5 minutes after birth.

C. To obtain an APGAR score, score 0, 1, or 2 for the five characteristics and add them together **(Table 21-1).**

1. An **APGAR score** of 0–3 indicates a life-threatening situation.

2. An **APGAR score** of 4–6 indicates that temperature and ventilation support is needed.

3. An **APGAR score** of 7–10 indicates a normal situation.

VII. PUERPERIUM extends from immediately after delivery of the baby until the reproductive tract returns to the nonpregnant state in approximately 4–6 weeks. Important events that occur follow.

A. Involution of the uterus occurs.

B. Afterpains occur, caused by uterine contractions.

C. Uterine discharge (**lochia**) occurs.

Table 21-1
Assessing the APGAR Score

Characteristic	Score			Example*
	0	**1**	**2**	**Example***
Appearance, color	Blue, pale	Body pink, extremities blue	Completely pink	1
Pulse, heart rate	Absent	< 100 bpm	> 100 bpm	2
Grimace, reflex, irritability	No response	Grimace	Vigorous crying	0
Activity, muscle tone	Flaccid	Some flexion of the extremities	Active motion, flexed extremities	0
Respiratory effort	None	Weak, irregular	Good, crying	1
APGAR Score				**4**

Clinical example: A newborn infant at 5 minutes after birth has a pink body but blue extremities (score 1); a heart rate of 125 bpm (score 2); shows no grimace or reflex (score 0); has flaccid muscle tone (score 0); has weak irregular breathing (score 1). The total APGAR score is 4. This infant needs ventilation and temperature support.

   D. In nonlactating women, ovulation returns 2–4 weeks postpartum and menstrual flow returns within 6–8 weeks postpartum.

   E. In lactating women, ovulation may return within 10 weeks postpartum. Birth control protection afforded by lactation is ensured for only 6 weeks, after which pregnancy is possible.

VIII. LACTATION

   A. During pregnancy, HPL, PRL, progesterone, estrogens, cortisol, and insulin stimulate the growth of **lactiferous ducts** and proliferation of epithelial cells to form **alveoli; alveoli secrete colostrum.**

   B. After delivery of the baby, **lactation (milk production)** is initiated by a decrease in progesterone and estrogens, along with the release of PRL from the adenohypophysis.

   C. During suckling, a stimulus from the breast inhibits the release of PRL-inhibiting factor from the hypothalamus, thus causing a **surge in PRL,** which increases milk production.

   D. Stimulation of the nipples during suckling causes a **surge of oxytocin,** which causes the **expulsion of accumulated milk (milk letdown)** by stimulating myoepithelial cells.

22

Numerical Chromosomal Abnormalities

I. POLYPLOIDY is the addition of extra haploid sets of chromosomes (i.e., 23) to the normal diploid set of chromosomes (i.e., 46).

  A. **Triploidy** is a condition in which cells contain **69 chromosomes.** It results in spontaneous abortion of the conceptus or only brief survival of the liveborn infant after birth. Triploidy occurs as a result of either a **failure of meiosis in a germ cell** (e.g., fertilization of a diploid egg by a haploid sperm) or **dispermy** (two sperm that fertilize one egg).

  B. **Tetraploidy** is a condition whereby cells contain **92 chromosomes.** It results in spontaneous abortion of the conceptus. Tetraploidy occurs as a result of **failure of the first cleavage division.**

II. ANEUPLOIDY is the addition of one chromosome (**trisomy**) or loss of one chromosome (**monosomy**). Trisomy usually results in spontaneous abortion of the conceptus; however, trisomy 13 (Patau's syndrome), trisomy 18 (Edwards' syndrome), trisomy 21 (Down syndrome), and Klinefelter's syndrome (47, XYY) are found in the liveborn population. Monosomy usually results in spontaneous abortion of the conceptus; however, monosomy X chromosome (45, X; Turner's syndrome) is found in the liveborn population. Aneuploidy occurs as a result of **nondisjunction during meiosis (Figure 22-1).**

  A. **Trisomy 13 (Patau's syndrome)** is characterized by profound mental retardation, congenital heart defects, cleft lip and palate, omphalocele, and polydactyly. Infants usually die soon after birth.

  B. **Trisomy 18 (Edwards' syndrome)** is characterized by mental retardation, congenital heart defects, small facies and prominent occiput, overlapping fingers, and rocker-bottom heels. Infants usually die soon after birth.

  C. **Trisomy 21, or Down syndrome (Figure 22-2 A–C),** is characterized by moderate mental retardation, microcephaly, microphthalmia, colobomata, cataracts and glaucoma, flat nasal bridge, epicanthic folds, protruding tongue, simian crease in the hand, and congenital heart defects. Alzheimer's neurofibrillary tangles and plaques are found in Down syndrome patients who are older than 30 years. Acute megakaryocytic leukemia (AMKL) is frequently present.

   1. This syndrome is the **most common type of trisomy;** its frequency increases with **advanced maternal age.**

   2. Trisomy 21 is associated with **low α-fetoprotein levels** in amniotic fluid or maternal serum.

   3. A specific region on chromosome 21 seems to be markedly associated with nu-

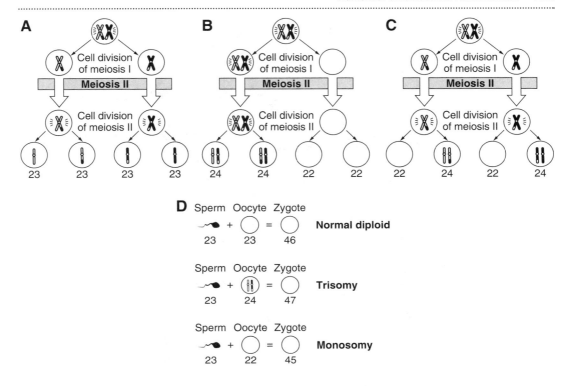

Figure 22-1.   (*A*) Normal meiotic divisions (I and II) producing gametes with 23 chromosomes. (*B*) Nondisjunction occurring in meiosis I produces gametes with 24 and 22 chromosomes. (*C*) Nondisjunction occurring in meiosis II produces gametes with 24 and 22 chromosomes. (*D*) Although nondisjunction may occur in either spermatogenesis or oogenesis, there is a higher frequency of nondisjunction in oogenesis. In this schematic, nondisjunction in oogenesis is depicted. If an abnormal oocyte (24 chromosomes) is fertilized by a normal sperm (23 chromosomes), a zygote with 47 chromosomes is produced (i.e., trisomy). If an abnormal oocyte (22 chromosomes) is fertilized by a normal sperm (23 chromosomes), a zygote with 45 chromosomes is produced (i.e., monosomy).

merous features of trisomy 21; this region is called **Down syndrome critical region (DSCR).** The following genes have been mapped to the DSCR (although their role is far from clear): carbonyl reductase, SIM2 (a transcription factor), p60 subunit of chromatin assembly factor, holocarboxylase synthetase, ERG (a proto-oncogene), GIRK2 (a potassium ion channel), and PEP19 (a calcium-dependent signal transducer.

4. Trisomy 21 may also be caused by a chromosomal **translocation** (see Chapter 23 III B) between chromosomes 14 and 21 [i.e., t(14;21)].

D. **Klinefelter's syndrome, or 47, XXY (Figure 22-2 D),** is a trisomic condition **found only in males** and characterized by hypogonadism, sterility, gynecomastia, elevated gonadotropin levels, and eunuchoid habitus.

E. **Turner's syndrome (monosomy X; 45,X; Figure 22-2 E)** is a monosomic condition

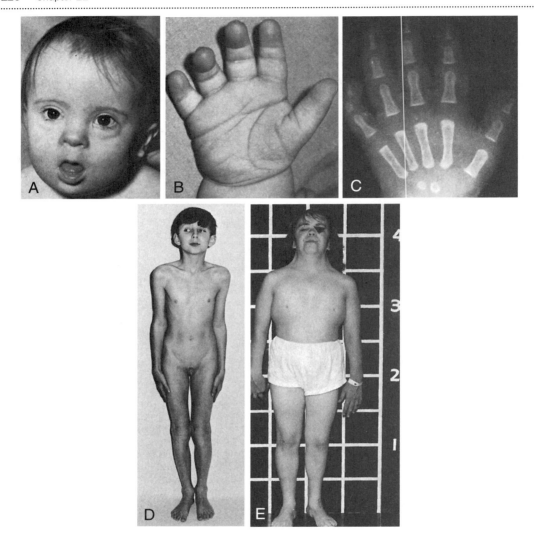

Figure 22-2. (A) An infant with Down syndrome. Note the flat nasal bridge, epicanthic folds, and protruding tongue. (B) Hand of a Down syndrome patient showing the simian crease. (C) Radiograph of hand in Down syndrome showing the curved fifth digit and malformation of the middle phalange of the fifth digit. (D) A 14-year-old boy with Klinefelter's syndrome (47,XXY). Note the hypogonadism and eunuchoid habitus. (E) A 14-year-old girl with Turner's syndrome (45,X). Note the webbed neck (due to delayed maturation of lymphatics), shield chest, and pinpoint nipples. (A, B, C, and E, from Smith DW, Jones KL: *Recognizable Patterns of Human Malformation*, 3rd ed. Philadelphia, WB Saunders, 1982, pp 13 and 75. D, from Salmon MA, Lindenbaum RH: *Developmental Defects and Syndromes*. Aylesbury, England, HM & M Publishers, 1978, p 372.)

found only in females and characterized by hypogonadism, congenital heart defects, webbed neck due to delayed maturation of lymphatics, shield chest, pinpoint nipples, edema of the hands and feet, aortic coarctation, ovarian fibrous streaks (i.e., infertility), and growth retardation. This syndrome is a common cause of **primary amenorrhea.**

23

Structural Chromosomal Abnormalities

I. DELETIONS are a loss of chromatin from a chromosome. The following are clinical examples caused by deletions.

    A. Chromosome 4p deletion (Wolf-Hirschhorn syndrome)

        1. Cause. Wolf-Hirschhorn syndrome is caused by a deletion in the short arm of chromosome 4 (4p); the specific region involved is **4p16.**

        2. Characteristics include a prominent forehead and broad nasal root (Greek "warrior helmet"), short philtrum, down-turned mouth, congenital heart defects, growth retardation, and severe mental retardation.

    B. Chromosome 5p deletion (cri du chat or cat's cry syndrome)

        1. Cause. Cri du chat syndrome is caused by a deletion in the short arm of chromosome 5 (5p); the specific region involved is **5p15.**

        2. Characteristics include a round facies, a cat-like cry, congenital heart defects, microcephaly, and mental retardation.

    C. Ring chromosome 14

        1. Cause. Ring chromosome 14 occurs when chromosome 14 forms a ring structure with breakpoints at **14p11** and **14q32.**

        2. Characteristics include mild dysmorphic features, frequent seizures, and variable mental retardation.

II. MICRODELETIONS are a loss of chromatin from a chromosome, which can be detected only by high-resolution banding. The following are clinical examples of syndromes caused by microdeletions.

    A. Prader-Willi syndrome

        1. Cause. Prader-Willi syndrome is caused by a microdeletion in the long arm of chromosome 15 (15q) derived from the **father (i.e., paternal imprinting);** the specific region involved is **15q11–13.**

        2. Characteristics include hyperphagia (insatiable appetite), hypogonadism, hypotonia, obesity, short stature, small hands and feet, behavior problems (rage, violence), and mild-to-moderate mental retardation.

        3. This syndrome is an example of **parental imprinting,** whereby the expression of certain genes derived from the father differs from the expression of the same genes derived from the mother. Parental imprinting occurs during gametogenesis due to

DNA methylation of cytosine nucleotides. Other examples of parental imprinting include **hydatidiform mole** (paternal imprinting) and **Beckwith-Wiedemann syndrome** (paternal imprinting).

4. The counterpart of Prader-Willi syndrome is Angelman's syndrome.

B. Angelman's syndrome (happy puppet syndrome)

1. Cause. Angelman's syndrome is caused by a microdeletion in the long arm of chromosome 15 (15q) derived from the **mother (i.e., maternal imprinting)**; the specific region involved is **15q11–13.**

2. Characteristics include gait ataxia (stiff, jerky, unsteady, upheld arms), seizures, happy disposition with inappropriate laughter, and severe mental retardation (only a 5–10 word vocabulary.)

3. This syndrome is another example of **parental imprinting** (see A 3).

4. The counterpart of Angelman's syndrome is Prader-Willi syndrome.

C. DiGeorge syndrome (DS)

1. Cause. DS is caused by a microdeletion in the long arm of chromosome 21 (21q); the specific region involved is **21q11 [also called the DGCR (DiGeorge chromosomal region)].**

2. Characteristics include congenital heart defects in the conotruncal region, immunodeficiency due to the absence of the thymus gland, hypocalcemia due to the absence of the parathyroid glands, hypertelorism, low-set prominent ears, and micrognathia.

3. DS has a phenotypic and genotypic similarity to **velocardiofacial syndrome (VCFS),** that is, both DS and VCFS are manifestations of a microdeletion at 21q11.

4. The following genes have been mapped to 21q11 or the DGCR (although their role is far from clear): catechol-O-methyltransferase (COMT; an enzyme used in catecholamine metabolism), GpIbb (receptor for von Willebrand factor), DGCR3 (a leucine zipper transcription factor), and citrate transport protein (CTP).

D. Miller-Dieker syndrome (agyria, lissencephaly)

1. Cause. Miller-Dieker syndrome is caused by a microdeletion in the short arm of chromosome 17; the specific region is **17p13.3.**

2. Characteristics include lissencephaly (smooth brain, i.e., no gyri), microcephaly, and a high and furrowing forehead. Death occurs at an early age.

3. Miller-Dieker syndrome should not be mistakenly diagnosed in the case of premature infants whose brains have not yet developed an adult pattern of gyri (gyri begin to appear normally at about week 28).

III. TRANSLOCATIONS result from breakage and exchange of segments between chromosomes. The following are clinical examples.

A. Robertsonian translocation t(13q14q)

1. Cause. This is a translocation between the long arms (q) of chromosomes 13 and 14 where the breakpoints are near the centromere; the short arms (p) of chromosomes 13 and 14 are generally lost.

2. Characteristics. Carriers of this Robertsonian translocation are **clinically normal**

because 13p and 14p, which are lost, contain only inert DNA and some rRNA (ribosomal RNA) genes that occur in multiple copies on other chromosomes.

3. This translocation is the **most common translocation found in humans.**

B. **Robertsonian translocation t(14q21q)**

  1. **Cause.** This is a translocation between the long arms (q) of chromosomes 14 and 21 where the breakpoints are near the centromere; the short arms (p) of chromosomes 14 and 21 are generally lost.

  2. **Characteristics.** Carriers of this Robertsonian translocation are **clinically normal.**

  3. The clinical issue in this translocation concerns reproduction. Depending on how the chromosomes segregate during meiosis, conception can produce offspring with trisomy 21 (livebirth), trisomy 14 (early miscarriage), monosomy 14 or 21 (early miscarriage), normal chromosome complement (live birth), or a t(14q21q) carrier (live birth). Consequently, in a couple where one member is a t(14q21q) carrier, the offspring may present with trisomy 21 (Down syndrome) or the woman may have recurrent miscarriages.

C. **Acute promyelocytic leukemia t(15;17)(q21;q21)**

  1. **Cause.** This disorder is caused by a reciprocal translocation between band q21 on chromosome 15 and band q21 on chromosome 17.

  2. **Result.** The result is a fusion of the **promyelocyte gene** (PML gene) on chromosome 15q21 with the **retinoic acid receptor gene (RARα gene)** on chromosome 17q21, thus forming the *pml/rarα* oncogene. The **PML/RARα oncoprotein** (a transcription factor) blocks the differentiation of promyelocytes to mature granulocytes such that there is continued proliferation of promyelocytes.

  3. **Characteristics** include coagulopathy and severe bleeding.

D. **Chronic myeloid leukemia t(9;22)(q34;q11)**

  1. **Cause.** This disorder is caused by a reciprocal translocation between band q34 on chromosome 9 and band q11 on chromosome 22; this is referred to as the **Philadelphia chromosome.**

  2. **Result.** The result is a fusion of the **ABL gene** on chromosome 9q34 with the **BCR gene** on chromosome 22q11, thus forming the *abl/bcr* oncogene. The **ABL/BCR oncoprotein** (a tyrosine kinase) has enhanced tyrosine kinase activity, which transforms hematopoietic precursor cells.

  3. **Characteristics** include an increased number of granulocytes in all stages of maturation and many mature neutrophils.

IV. **FRAGILE SITES** are gaps or breaks in chromosomes that can be visualized if cell cultures are exposed to specific culture conditions. **Fragile X syndrome (Martin-Bell syndrome),** described below, is one clinical example.

A. **Cause.** Fragile X syndrome is caused by a fragile site on chromosome X; the specific region involved is **Xq27.**

B. **Characteristics** include macroorchidism, speech delay, behavioral problems (e.g., hyperactivity, attention deficit), prominent jaw, and large, dysmorphic ears.

C. The fragile site is observed when cells are cultured in a **folate-depleted** medium. The fragile site is produced by a **trinucleotide (CGG) repeat mutation** in the **FMR1 gene.** The FMR1 gene encodes for a protein called **FMRP,** whose exact function is unknown but has RNA-binding capability.

D. This syndrome is the **leading cause of inherited mental retardation** (most severe in males).

V. ISOCHROMOSOMES occur when the centromere divides transversely (instead of longitudinally) such that one of the chromosome arms is duplicated and the other arm is lost. **Isochromosome Xq,** described below, is one clinical example.

   A. Cause. Isochromosome Xq is a duplication of the long arm(q) and loss of the short arm (p) of chromosome X.

   B. This isochromosome is found in 20% of females with **Turner's syndrome** (see Chapter 22 II E).

   C. The occurrence of isochromosomes within any of the autosomes is generally lethal.

VI. INVERSIONS are the reversal of the order of DNA between two breaks in a chromosome.

   A. Pericentric inversions occur on both sides of the centromere; **paracentric inversions** occur on the same side of the centromere.

   B. Carriers of inversions are normal.

   C. Diagnosis is generally a coincidental finding during prenatal testing or the repeated occurrence of spontaneous abortions or stillbirths.

VII. BREAKAGE. Breaks in chromosomes are caused by sunlight or ultraviolet irradiation, ionizing irradiation, DNA cross-linking agents, or DNA-damaging agents. These insults may cause **depurination of DNA, deamination of cytosine to uracil,** or **pyrimidine dimerization,** which must be repaired by DNA repair enzymes. The clinical importance of DNA repair enzymes is illustrated by some rare inherited diseases that involve genetic defects in DNA repair enzymes, such as the following.

   A. Xeroderma pigmentosum (XP) is a genetic skin disease in which the affected individuals are hypersensitive to **sunlight (ultraviolet radiation).**

   1. Cause. XP is caused by a genetic defect in one or more of the enzymes involved in the removal of pyrimidine dimers, which in humans have been shown to require at least eight different gene products.

   2. Characteristics include severe skin lesions and malignant skin cancer; most affected individuals die by 30 years of age.

   B. Ataxia-telangiectasia is a genetic disease in which the affected individual is hypersensitive to **ionizing radiation.**

   1. Cause. Ataxia-telangiectasia is caused by genetic defects in enzymes involved in DNA repair.

   2. Characteristics include cerebellar ataxia, oculocutaneous telangiectasia, and immunodeficiency.

   C. Fanconi's anemia is a genetic disease in which affected individuals are hypersensitive to DNA cross-linking agents.

   1. Cause. Fanconi's anemia is caused by genetic defects in enzymes involved in DNA repair.

   2. Characteristics include leukemia and progressive aplastic anemia.

   D. Bloom's syndrome is a genetic disease in which affected individuals are hypersensitive to a **wide variety of DNA-damaging agents.**

1. Cause. Bloom's syndrome is caused by widespread genetic defects in enzymes involved in DNA repair.

2. Characteristics include immunodeficiency, growth retardation, and predisposition to several types of cancers.

E. Hereditary nonpolyposis colorectal cancer (HNPCC). Although most colorectal cancers are not genetic diseases, HPNCC accounts for **15% of all cases of colorectal cancer.**

1. The genes involved in HPNCC have been identified as **MSH2 genes.** The MSH2 genes are the human homologues to the *Escherichia coli* **mutS** and **mutL** genes that code for DNA repair enzymes.

2. Identification of the genes responsible for HPNCC allows individuals at risk for this inherited cancer to be identified by genetic testing. Early diagnosis greatly improves the chances of patient survival, because the early stage of this disease is the outgrowth of small benign polyps that can be removed easily by surgery before malignancy.

VIII. SELECTED PHOTOMICROGRAPHS

A. Chromosome 4P deletion (Woilf-Hirschhorn syndrome) and chromosome 5p deletion (cri-du-chat syndrome: **Figure 23-1**

B. Prader-Willi syndrome, Angelman's syndrome, DiGeorge syndrome, Miller-Dieker syndrome: **Figure 23-2**

C. Robertsonian t(13q14q), Robertsonian t(14q21q), acute promyelocytic leukemia t (15;17)(q21;q21), chronic myeloid leukemia t(9;22)(q34;q11): **Figure 23-3**

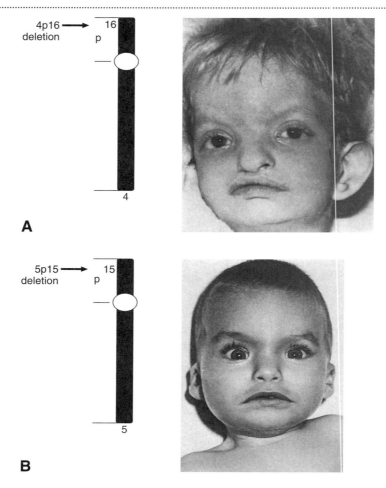

Figure 23-1. Deletion abnormalities. (*A*) Chromosome 4p deletion (Wolf-Hirschhorn syndrome). The deletion at 4p16 is shown on chromosome 4. The photograph of a 5-year-old boy with Wolf-Hirschhorn syndrome reveals a prominent forehead and broad nasal root (Greek "warrior helmet"), short philtrum, and down-turned mouth; severe mental retardation (IQ = 20) is a characteristic of this syndrome. (*B*) Chromosome 5p deletion (cri du chat syndrome or cat's cry syndrome). The deletion at 5p15 is shown on chromosome 5. The photograph of an infant with cri du chat syndrome shows round facies and microcephaly; this defect also causes mental retardation. (Photo in *A* from Smith DW, Jones KL: *Recognizable Patterns of Human Malformation*, 3rd ed. Philadelphia, WB Saunders, 1982, p 37. Photo in *B* from Salmon MA, Lindenbaum RH: *Developmental Defects and Syndromes*. Aylesbury, England, HM & M Publishers, 1978, p 321.)

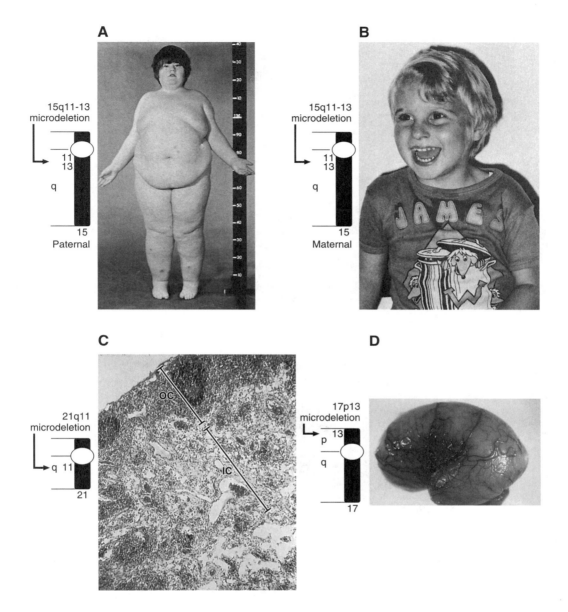

Figure 23-2. Microdeletion abnormalities. (A) Prader-Willi syndrome. The microdeletion at 15q11–13 is shown on chromosome 15, which was inherited from the father (paternal). The photograph of a 10-year-old boy with Prader-Willi syndrome shows hypogonadism, hypotonia, obesity, short stature, and small hands and feet. (B) Angelman's syndrome (happy puppet syndrome). The microdeletion at 15q11–13 is shown on chromosome 15, which was inherited from the mother (maternal). The photograph of a 5-year-old boy with Angelman's syndrome shows the boy's happy disposition; the syndrome is characterized by inappropriate laughter and severe mental retardation (with only a 5–10 word vocabulary). (C) DiGeorge syndrome. The microdeletion at 21q11 is shown on chromosome 21. The photomicrograph of a lymph node from a patient with DiGeorge syndrome shows the absence of T lymphocytes within the inner cortex (*IC*, paracortex, or thymic-dependent zone). The outer cortex (*OC*) shows abundant B lymphocytes within lymphatic follicles. (D) Miller-Dieker syndrome (agyria, lissencephaly). The microdeletion at 17p13 is shown on chromosome 17. The photograph of a brain at autopsy from an infant with Miller-Dieker syndrome shows the complete absence of gyri. (A and B, from Salmon MA, Lindenbaum RH: *Developmental Defects and Syndromes*. Aylesbury, England, HM & M Publishers, 1978, pp 139 and 169. C and D, from Gilbert-Barness E: *Potter's Atlas of Fetal and Infant Pathology*. St Louis, CV Mosby, 1998, pp 254 and 277.)

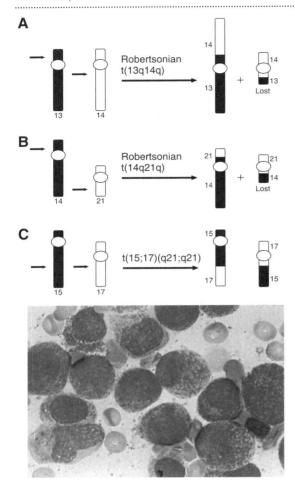

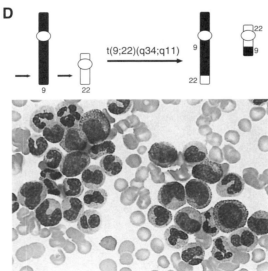

Figure 23-3. Translocation abnormalities. (A) Robertsonian t(13q14q). (B) Robertsonian t(14q21q). (C) Acute promyelocytic leukemia t(15;17)(q21;q21). The translocation between chromosomes 15 and 17 is shown forming the pml/rarα oncogene. The photomicrograph of acute promyelocytic leukemia shows abnormal promyelocytes with their characteristic pattern of heavy granulation and bundle of Auer rods. (D) Chronic myeloid leukemia t(9;22)(q34;q11). The translocation between chromosomes 9 and 22 is shown forming the Philadelphia chromosome with the abl/bcr oncogene. The photomicrograph of chronic myeloid leukemia shows marked granulocytic hyperplasia with neutrophilic precursors at all stages of maturation. Erythroid (red blood cell) precursors are significantly decreased; none are shown in this field. (C and D, from Mufti GJ, Flandrin G, Schaefer HE et al: *An Atlas of Malignant Haematology.* Philadelphia, Lippincott-Raven, 1996, pp 73 and 179.)

24

Single Gene Inherited Diseases

I. AUTOSOMAL DOMINANT INHERITANCE

A. Introduction. Diseases that have autosomal dominant inheritance affect individuals who receive only one defective copy of the gene from either parent. An example of an autosomal dominant inherited disease is Huntington's disease (HD). Other autosomal dominant inherited disorders are listed in the Appendix.

B. Huntington disease (HD)

1. The characteristic dysfunction is the **cell death of cholinergic neurons and GABA-ergic neurons** within the **caudate nucleus** (corpus striatum). This results clinically in **choreic (dance-like) movements, mood disturbances, and progressive loss of mental activity.** No treatment is available.

2. HD is caused by **autosomal dominant mutation** so that an individual need receive only one defective copy of the HD gene to have the disease.

3. The HD gene is located on the **short arm (p arm) of chromosome 4 (4p).**

4. The HD gene encodes for a protein that has yet to be identified.

5. The mechanism for neuronal cell death in Huntington's disease may involve a **hyperactive N-methyl-D-aspartate (NMDA) receptor** as indicated below:
   a. Because glutamate is the main excitatory transmitter in the brain, almost all neurons have **glutamate receptors,** one of which is called the **NMDA receptor.** The NMDA receptor is so named because it is selectively activated by the glutamate agonist called **NMDA.**
   b. In normal synaptic transmission, glutamate levels rise transiently within the synaptic cleft. However, excessive and diffuse release of glutamate results in neuronal cell death called **glutamate toxicity.**
   c. Glutamate toxicity is the result of an **excessive influx of calcium into the neurons** because of the sustained action of glutamate on the NMDA receptor.
   d. It is thought that the mutation of the HD gene on 4p somehow results in a **hyperactive NMDA receptor** so that excessive influx of calcium into neurons of the caudate nucleus occurs with resultant cell death.

II. AUTOSOMAL RECESSIVE INHERITANCE

A. Introduction. Diseases that have autosomal recessive inheritance affect only individuals who receive two copies of the gene (one from each parent). An example of an autosomal recessive inherited disease is cystic fibrosis (CF). Other autosomal recessive diseases are listed in Appendix A.

B. Cystic fibrosis (CF)

1. The characteristic dysfunction in CF is the **production of abnormally thick mucus** by epithelial cells lining the respiratory and gastrointestinal tracts. This results clinically in **obstruction of pulmonary airways and recurrent respiratory bacterial infections.**

2. CF is caused by **autosomal recessive mutation** such that an individual must receive two defective copies of the CF gene (one from each parent) to have the disease.

3. The CF gene is located on the **long arm (q arm) of chromosome 7 (7q)** between bands q21 and q31.

4. The CF gene encodes for a protein called cystic fibrosis transporter **(CFTR),** which functions as a **Cl^- ion channel.**

5. A mutation in the CF gene destroys the Cl^- transport function of CFTR.

6. In North America, 70% of cystic fibrosis cases are caused by a **three-base deletion** that codes for the amino acid **phenylalanine at position 508** so that phenylalanine is missing from CFTR.

III. X-LINKED RECESSIVE INHERITANCE

A. Introduction

1. In X-linked recessive inheritance, the disease is usually observed only in the male, because males have only one X chromosome, that is, males are **hemizygous** for X-linked genes (i.e., there is no backup copy of the gene). In X-linked recessive inheritance, heterozygous females are clinically normal but the trait may be detected by subtle clinical features (e.g., intermediate enzyme levels).

2. Can the disease ever be observed in females? The answer is affirmative according to the following mechanism: In females, one of the two X chromosomes is inactivated during the **late blastocyst stage** to form a **Barr body** in a process called **dosage compensation.** The choice of whether the maternally derived or paternally derived X chromosome is deactivated is a **random and permanent event.** The mechanism of dosage compensation involves **methylation of cytosine nucleotides.** If the X chromosome with the normal gene is deactivated, the female has one X chromosome with the abnormal gene and will, therefore, be affected by the disease.

3. An example of X-linked recessive inherited disease is Duchenne muscular dystrophy (DMD). Other examples are listed in Appendix A.

B. Duchenne muscular dystrophy (DMD)

1. The characteristic dysfunction in DMD is **progressive muscle weakness and wasting.** This results clinically in **premature death due to cardiac or respiratory failure** in persons in their late teens to 20s.

2. DMD is caused by **X-linked recessive mutation** so that the male need only receive one defective copy of the DMD gene (from the mother) to have the disease.

3. The DMD gene is located on the **short arm (p arm) of chromosome X in band 21 (Xp21).**

4. The DMD gene encodes for a protein called **dystrophin,** which anchors the cytoskeleton (actin) of skeletal muscle cells to the extracellular matrix via a transmembrane protein (α-dystroglycan and β-dystroglycan), thus stabilizing the cell membrane.

5. A mutation of the DMD gene destroys the ability of dystrophin to anchor actin to the extracellular matrix.

IV. MITOCHONDRIAL INHERITANCE

A. Introduction. Diseases that have mitochondrial inheritance are caused by mutations in the mitochondrial DNA (mtDNA). They are inherited entirely through **maternal transmission** because sperm mitochondria do not pass into the ovum at fertilization. An example of a mitochondrial inherited disease is Leber hereditary optic neuropathy (LHON). Other examples are listed in Appendix A.

B. Leber hereditary optic neuropathy (LHON)

1. The characteristic dysfunction in LHON is **progressive optic nerve degeneration.** This results clinically in **blindness.**

2. Of all cases of LHON, 50% involve the **ND4 gene** located on mtDNA when a missense mutation changes **arginine to histidine.**

3. The ND4 gene encodes for a protein called **subunit 4 of the NADH dehydroge-**

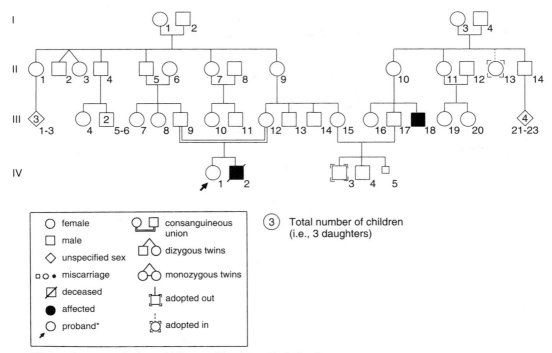

Figure 24-1. Family pedigree and explanation of the various symbols. (Modified from Friedman JM, Dill FJ, Hayden MR, McGillivray BC: *Genetics*. Malvern, PA, Williams & Wilkins, 1992, p 151.)

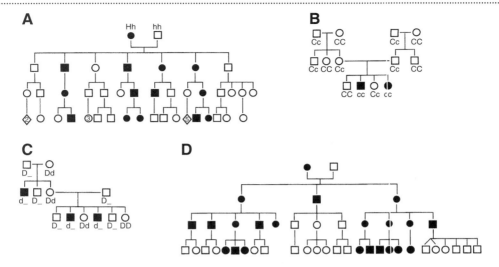

Figure 24-2. (A) Pedigree of autosomal dominant inheritance. (Huntington disease) (B) Pedigree of autosomal recessive inheritance. (cystic fibrosis) (C) Pedigree of X-linked recessive inheritance. (Duchenne muscular dystrophy) Note that the three affected males are siblings of unaffected mothers. (D) Pedigree of mitochondrial inheritance. (Leber hereditary optic neuropathy) Note that affected sons and daughters are siblings of an affected mother, and affected fathers do not produce affected siblings. (A–D, modified from Dudek RW: *High-Yield Cell and Molecular Biology.* Philadelphia, Lippincott Williams & Wilkins, 1999, pp 64, 65, 67, 68.)

nase complex, which functions in the **electron transport chain** and the **production of ATP.**

4. A mutation of the ND4 gene decreases the production of ATP with the result that the demands of a very active neuronal metabolism cannot be met.

V. FAMILY PEDIGREE is a graphic method of charting the family history using various symbols **(Figure 24-1).** Family pedigrees of various inherited diseases are shown in **Figure 24-2.**

25

Multifactorial Inherited Diseases

I. INTRODUCTION. Multifactorial inheritance involves many genes that have a small, equal, and additive effect (**genetic component**) as well as an **environmental component.** Both components contribute to a person inheriting the liability to develop a certain disease. If one considers only the genetic component of a multifactorial disease, the term **polygenic** is used. An example of a multifactorial disease is Type I diabetes; others are listed in the Appendix.

II. TYPE I DIABETES

    A. The characteristic dysfunction is the **destruction of pancreatic beta cells** that produce insulin. This results clinically in hyperglycemia, ketoacidosis, and exogenous insulin dependence. Long-term clinical effects include neuropathy, retinopathy leading to blindness, and nephropathy leading to kidney failure.

    B. Type I diabetes demonstrates an association with the highly polymorphic **human leukocyte antigen (HLA) class II genes** that play a role in the immune response. The specific loci involved in Type I diabetes are called **HLA-DR3** and **HLA-DR4 loci;** they are located on the **short arm (p arm) of chromosome 6 (p6).**

    C. HLA-DR3 and HLA-DR4 are loci code for **cell surface glycoproteins** that are structurally similar to immunoglobulin proteins and are expressed mainly by B lymphocytes and macrophages.

    D. It is *hypothesized* that alleles closely linked to HLA-DR3 and HLA-DR4 loci somehow alter the immune response so that the individual has an immune response to an environmental antigen (e.g., virus). The immune response "spills over" and leads to the destruction of pancreatic beta cells.

    E. Markers for immune destruction of pancreatic beta cells include **autoantibodies to glutamic acid decarboxylase (GAD_{65}), insulin,** and **tyrosine phosphatases IA-2 and IA-2β.** At present, it is unknown whether the autoantibodies play a causative role in the destruction of the pancreatic beta cells or the autoantibodies form secondarily after the pancreatic beta cells have been destroyed.

26
Teratology

I. INTRODUCTION. A **teratogen** is any infectious agent, drug, chemical, or irradiation that alters fetal morphology or fetal function if the fetus is exposed during a critical stage of development.

A. The **resistant period (week 1 of development)** is the time when the conceptus demonstrates the "all-or-none" phenomenon (i.e., the conceptus will either die as a result of the teratogen or survive unaffected).

B. The **maximum susceptibility period (weeks 3–8; embryonic period)** is the time when the embryo is most susceptible to teratogens, because all organ morphogenesis occurs at this time.

C. The **lowered susceptibility period (weeks 9–38; fetal period)** is the time when the fetus has a lowered susceptibility to teratogens, because all organs systems have already formed. The result of teratogen exposure during this period is generally the *functional* derangement of an organ system.

II. INFECTIOUS AGENTS may be viral or nonviral; however, bacteria appear to be nonteratogenic.

A. Viral infections may reach the fetus via the amniotic fluid following vaginal infection, transplacentally via the bloodstream after maternal viremia, or by direct contact during passage through an infected birth canal.

1. Rubella virus (German measles) infection during pregnancy can cause the classic triad of fetal **cardiac defects:** patent ductus arteriosus, pulmonary artery stenosis, and atrioventricular (AV) septal defects. It also causes **cataracts** and **deafness.**

2. Cytomegalovirus (CMV), a ubiquitous virus and the most common fetal infection, is the cause of **cytomegalic inclusion disease,** which affects primarily the central nervous system.

a. CMV results in microcephaly, chorioretinitis, hepatosplenomegaly, cerebral calcification, mental retardation, heart block, and petechiae.

b. The risk of malformations is much higher in infants of mothers who had a primary CMV infection during pregnancy compared with mothers who have had recurrent infections.

3. Herpes virus type 2 (HSV-2) is transmitted by maternal viremia or by direct contact during passage through an infected birth canal.

a. Although herpetic infections are quite common in women, transmission of maternal HSV-2 to the fetus is uncommon (i.e., < 1 in 7500 cases).

b. HSV-2 rarely causes fetal malformations.

    c. HSV-2 may result in fetal growth retardation, microcephaly, chorioretinitis, and cerebral calcification

  4. **Varicella zoster virus (VZV; chickenpox)** is transmitted to the fetus, in 24% of the cases, following maternal varicella infection during the last month of pregnancy. VZV results in fetal skin scarring, limb hypoplasia, rudimentary digits, club foot, microcephaly, and mental retardation.

  5. **Human immunodeficiency virus (HIV)** is believed by some to cause **acquired immunodeficiency syndrome (AIDS).** HIV does not cause any congenital malformation.

B. **Nonviral infections**

  1. *Toxoplasma gondii* is a **protozoan parasite** that is found particularly in **cats.** It is transmitted to the fetus transplacentally. *T. gondii* may cause miscarriage, perinatal death, chorioretinitis, microcephaly, and cerebral calcification.

  2. *Treponema pallidum* is a **spirochete** that causes **syphilis.** It is transmitted to the fetus transplacentally. This spirochete can cause miscarriage, perinatal death, hepatosplenomegaly, joint swelling, skin rash, anemia, jaundice, metaphyseal dystrophy, abnormal teeth (Hutchinson teeth), and changes in cerebrospinal fluid. Antibiotics given to the affected mother usually provide adequate therapy for the fetus.

III. CATEGORY X DRUGS (ABSOLUTE CONTRAINDICATION IN PREGNANCY)

A. **Thalidomide** is an **antinausea** drug that was at one time prescribed for pregnant women for "morning sickness." (It is no longer used.) This drug can cause fetal limb reduction (e.g., meromelia, amelia), ear and nasal abnormalities, cardiac defects, lung defects, pyloric or duodenal stenosis, and gastrointestinal atresia.

B. **Aminopterin and methotrexate** are **folic acid antagonists** used in cancer chemotherapy. If used during pregnancy, these drugs can result in small stature, abnormal cranial ossification, ocular hypertelorism, low-set ears, cleft palate, and myelomeningoceles.

C. **Busulfan (Myleran), chlorambucil (Leukeran), and cyclophosphamide (Cytoxan)** are **alkylating agents** used in cancer chemotherapy. Consumption during pregnancy may cause fetal cleft palate, eye defects, hydronephrosis, renal agenesis, absence of toes, and growth retardation.

D. **Phenytoin (Dilantin)** is an **antiepileptic** drug.

  1. In 30% of cases, consumption of phenytoin during pregnancy results in **fetal hydantoin syndrome,** which includes growth retardation, mental retardation, microcephaly, craniofacial defects, and nail and digit hypoplasia.

  2. In the majority of cases, consumption during pregnancy results in fetal cleft lip, cleft palate, and congenital heart defects.

E. **Triazolam (Halcion) and estazolam (ProSom)** are **hypnotic** drugs. Consumption during pregnancy, especially in the first trimester, results in fetal cleft lip and cleft palate.

F. **Warfarin (Coumadin)** is an **anticoagulant** drug that acts by inhibiting vitamin K–dependent coagulation factors. Use during pregnancy can cause stippled epiphyses, mental retardation, microcephaly, seizures, fetal hemorrhage, and optic atrophy in the fetus.

G. **Isotretinoin (Accutane)** is a **retinoic acid derivative** that is used to treat **severe acne.** Use during pregnancy can cause fetal CNS abnormalities, external ear abnormalities, eye abnormalities, facial dysmorphia, and cleft palate (i.e., **vitamin A embryopathy**).

H. **Clomiphene (Clomid)** is a nonsteroidal **ovulatory stimulant** that is used in women with ovulatory dysfunction. Although no causative evidence of a deleterious effect of clomiphene on the human fetus has been established, there have been reports of birth anomalies.

I. **Diethylstilbestrol** is a **synthetic estrogen** that was used to prevent spontaneous abortion in women. Many women who were exposed to DES in utero have reproductive system disorders including cervical hood, T-shaped uterus, hypoplastic uterus, ovulatory disorders, infertility, premature labor, and cervical incompetence. These women are also subject to **increased risk of adenocarcinoma of the vagina** later in life.

J. **Ethisterone, norethisterone, and megestrol (Megace)** are synthetic **progesterone derivatives.** Consumption during pregnancy results in masculinization of genitalia in female embryos, hypospadias in males, and cardiovascular anomalies.

K. **Ovcon, Levlen, and Norinyl** are **oral contraceptives** that contain a combination of estrogen (e.g., ethinyl estradiol or mestranol) and progesterone (e.g., norethindrone or levonorgestrel) derivatives. Consumption of these drugs during pregnancy results in an increase of fetal abnormalities, particularly the **VACTERL syndrome,** which consists of vertebral, anal, cardiac, tracheoesophageal, renal, and limb malformations.

L. **Nicotine** is a **poisonous, additive alkaloid** delivered to the fetus through **cigarette smoking** by pregnant women. (Cigarette smoke also contains **hydrogen cyanide** and **carbon monoxide.**) Smoking during pregnancy can cause intrauterine growth retardation, premature delivery, low birth weight, fetal hypoxia due to reduced uterine blood flow, and diminished capacity of the blood to transport oxygen to fetal tissue.

M. **Alcohol** is an **organic compound** delivered to the fetus through **recreational drinking or addictive drinking (i.e., alcoholism)** by pregnant women. Consumption of alcohol during pregnancy can cause **fetal alcohol syndrome,** which includes mental retardation, microcephaly, holoprosencephaly, limb deformities, craniofacial abnormalities (i.e., hypertelorism, long philtrum, and short palpebral fissures), and cardiovascular defects (i.e., ventricular septal defects). Fetal alcohol syndrome is the **leading cause of mental retardation.**

IV. CATEGORY D DRUGS (DEFINITE EVIDENCE OF RISK TO FETUS)

A. **Tetracycline (Achromycin) and doxycycline (Vibramycin)** are **antibiotics** in the tetracycline family. Use of these drugs during pregnancy results in permanently stained teeth and hypoplasia of enamel in the fetus.

B. **Streptomycin, amikacin, and tobramycin (Nebcin)** are **antibiotics** in the aminoglycoside family. Consumption of these drugs during pregnancy results in fetal **cranial nerve VIII toxicity** with permanent bilateral deafness and loss of vestibular function.

C. **Phenobarbital (Donnatal) and pentobarbital (Nembutal)** are **barbiturates** that are used as **sedatives.** Studies have suggested a higher incidence of fetal abnormalities with maternal barbiturate use.

D. **Valproic acid (Depakene)** is an **antiepileptic** drug. Consumption during pregnancy results in fetal neural tube defects, cleft lip, and renal defects.

E. **Diazepam (Valium), chlordiazepoxide (Librium), alprazolam (Xanax), and lorazepam (Ativan)** are **anticonvulsant** or **antianxiety** drugs. Consumption during pregnancy results in fetal cleft lip and cleft palate, especially if the drugs are used in the first trimester of pregnancy.

F. **Lithium** is used in the treatment of **manic-depressive disorder.** Consumption during pregnancy results in fetal cardiac defects (i.e., Ebstein anomaly and malformations of the great vessels).

G. Chlorothiazide (Diuril) is a **diuretic** and **antihypertensive** drug. Consumption during pregnancy results in fetal jaundice and thrombocytopenia.

V. CHEMICAL AGENTS

A. **Organic mercury.** Consumption of organic mercury during pregnancy results in fetal neurologic damage, including seizures, psychomotor retardation, cerebral palsy, blindness, and deafness.

B. **Lead.** Consumption of lead during pregnancy may result in abortion due to embryotoxicity, or it may cause fetal growth retardation, increased perinatal mortality, and developmental delay.

C. **Polychlorinated biphenyls (PCBs).** Consumption of PCBs during pregnancy results in intrauterine growth retardation, dark brown skin pigmentation, exophthalmos, gingival hyperplasia, skull calcification, mental retardation, and neurobehavioral abnormalities.

D. **Potassium iodide** is found in over-the-counter cough medicines and x-ray cocktails for organ visualization. Consumption during pregnancy results in fetal thyroid enlargement (goiter) and mental retardation (cretinism).

VI. RECREATIONAL DRUGS

A. **Lysergic acid diethylamide (LSD)** has not been shown to be teratogenic.

B. **Marijuana** has not been shown to be teratogenic.

C. **Caffeine** has not been shown to be teratogenic.

D. **Cocaine** consumption during pregnancy results in an increased risk of various congenital abnormalities, stillbirths, low birth weight, and placental abruption.

E. **Heroin** itself has not been shown to be teratogenic; it is the drugs that are often taken with heroin that produce congenital anomalies. The main adverse effect of heroin is **severe neonatal withdrawal,** which results in death in 3%–5% of neonates born to mothers addicted to heroin. **Methadone** (used to replace heroin) is not teratogenic but, like heroin, is associated with severe neonatal withdrawal.

VII. IONIZING RADIATION

A. **Acute high dose radiation (> 250 rads).** An acute overdose of ionizing radiation during pregnancy can cause fetal microcephaly, mental retardation, growth retardation, and leukemia. After exposure to **more than 25 rads,** classic fetal defects will be observed; termination of pregnancy should be offered as an option. Much information concerning acute high-dose radiation has come from studies of the atomic explosions over Hiroshima and Nagasaki.

B. **Diagnostic radiation.** Even if several x-ray studies are performed during pregnancy, rarely does the dose add up to significant exposure to produce fetal defects. **Radioactive iodine cocktails** for organ visualization **should be avoided after week 10** of gestation, because fetal thyroid development can be impaired.

Appendix

Inherited Diseases by Type

Autosomal Dominant	Autosomal Recessive	X-linked	Mitochondrial	Multifactorial
α₁-Antitrypsin	α-Thalassemia	**Recessive**	Cardiac rhythm disturbance?	Cancer
Achondroplasia	Adrenogenital syndrome	Duchenne type muscular	Cardiomyopathy?	Cleft lip
Actocephalosyndactyly	Albinism	dystrophy	Infantile bilateral striated	Cleft palate
Adult polycystic kidney	Alkaptonuria	Ectodermal dysplasia	necrosis	Clubfoot
disease	Ataxia telangiectasia	Fabry's disease	Kearns-Sayre syndrome	Congenital heart defect
Alport's syndrome	β-Thalassemia	Fragile X syndrome	Leber's hereditary optic	Coronary artery disease
Bor syndrome	Branched chain ketonuria	Hemophilia A and B	neuropathy	Epilepsy
Brachydactyly	Cystic fibrosis	Hunter's syndrome types		Hemochromatosis
Cleidocranial dysplasia	Cystinuria	A and B		Hirschsprung's disease
Craniostenosis	Dwarfism	Ichthyosis		Hyperlipoproteinemia types I,
Crouzon's disease	Erythropoietic porphyria	Kennedy's syndrome		IIb, III, IV, V
Diabetes associated with	Friedreich's ataxia	Kinky-hair syndrome		Hypertension
defects in the genes	Galactosemia	Lesch-Nyhan syndrome		Legg-Calve-Perthes disease
for glucokinase,	Glycogen storage disease	Leukocyte G-6-PD deficiency		Pyloric stenosis
HNF-1α, and HNF-4α	Hemoglobin C disease	Testicular feminization		Rheumatic fever
Ehlers-Danlos syndrome	Hepatolenticular	Wiskott-Aldrich syndrome		Type I diabetes
Epidermolysis bullosa	degeneration			(associated with islet
Familial	Histidinemia	**Dominant**		cell antibodies)
hypercholesterolemia	Homocystinuria	Goltz-syndrome		Type II diabetes
(type IIa)	Hypophosphatasia	Hypophosphatemic rickets		(associated with insulin
Goldenhar's syndrome	Hypothyroidism	Incontinentia pigmenti		resistance and obesity)
Heart-hand syndrome	Infantile polycystic kidney	Orofaciodigital syndrome		
Hereditary spherocytosis	disease			
Huntington's disease	Laurence-Moon syndrome			
Marfan syndrome	Lipidosis			
Myotonic dystrophy	Mucolipidosis			
Neurofibromatosis	Mucopolysaccharidosis			
Noonan's syndrome	Peroxisomal disorders			
Osteogenesis imperfecta	Phenylketonuria			
Treacher Collins syndrome	Premature senility			
von Willebrand's disease	Pyruvate kinase deficiency			
Waardenburg's syndrome	Retinitis pigmentosa			
Williams-Beuren syndrome	Sickle cell anemia			
	Tyrosinemia			

HNF = hepatocyte nuclear factor.
From Dudek RW: *High Yield Cell and Molecular Biology*. Philadelphia, Lippincott Williams & Wilkins, 1999; p 70.

Index

References in *italics* indicate figures; those followed by "t" denote tables